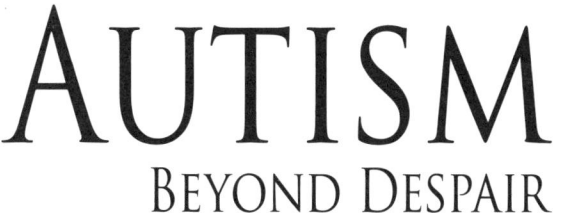

AUTISM
BEYOND DESPAIR

AUTISM
BEYOND DESPAIR

CEASE THERAPY

Homeopathy has the answers

Tinus Smits M.D.
Edited by Tim Owens

Enquiries should be addressed to:
Emryss Publishers
Email: info@emryss.com

First edition March 2010
Second Edition 2018
Third edtion 2020

© Dr. Tinus Smits
www.emryss.com

Edited by Tim Owens
Layout: Olivier Bakker
Cover design: Cheryl Feng
ISBN/EAN: 978-90-76189-28-4
NUR. 873
Access code: Homoeopathy, General health science, Autism

The birth of a healthy child is a miracle;

keeping a child healthy is an art.

Tinus Smits, M.D.

DISCLAIMER

Although this book discusses the homeopathic method of treatment, including stories of cure using various remedies, it is intended only as general introduction to the CEASE Therapy. This book is not intended to replace the services of qualified practitioners in the field. Any application of the recommendations set forth in the following pages is at the reader's discretion and sole risk. For those who want to have their children treated according to the CEASE therapy we recommend working with an experienced homeopath who is certified as a CEASE therapist. A list of such practitioners is available at www.cease-autism.com

ACKNOWLEDGEMENT

Gratitude is the feeling I have now that this book has come to publication. Gratitude that it could be completed in a relatively short time in order that the good news can now be spread to so many desperate parents of children with autism and behavioral problems. I am especially grateful for all those who have substantially contributed to make this a book of high interest.

First of all I want to thank Marie-Pierre, my wife, who had to tolerate my working like a workaholic in my practice and then spending most of my free time writing.

A special hug for my son Yannick, who has lightened my load in many ways during the birth process of the CEASE therapy by doing much of the organization and all of the computer work. He wants to dedicate his life to propagating the CEASE therapy. Thank you so much for grasping in such an early state the importance of this work. I am proud of you and I know you are proud of me. You are a fantastic boy.

Then I do not know how to thank my two editors who did a tremendous job preparing my English for publication. Thanks so much, Tim Owens, a homeopath from upstate New York as well as an English teacher with a feeling for literary matters. Tim completed my five day initiation course of Inspiring Homeopathy in France several summers ago. That makes him the ideal person to edit my book. Thank you, Tim; you have done a great job. And with him I want to thank my other editor, a professional editor and homeopath who prefers to remain anonymous. She has done a fantastic job of advising me about how to make this material understandable to parents, to doctors, and to homeopaths outside of Europe. She tempered me when at times I was a little too enthusiastic or too fanatic. I remember she once said, 'If you say that, you will lose the last regular doctor that still believes in you.' Thank you so much for your work and dedication. You both are people who live life in a conscious way and have chosen to bring about more happiness in this world.

I also want to thank Olivier Bakker from Emryss Publishing & Distribution, who has his heart in the right place. Meeting him was a real pleasure. He is young and dynamic, and I immediately had the feeling that he was the right person to publish such a book. He never put me under pressure to finish it earlier, and he patiently accepted the many delays brought on by my busy schedule. He just said: 'Tinus, take your time.'

And let me not forget the more than 80 certified CEASE therapists, who are now able to apply this wonderful method to heal autism. Their enthusiasm and high level of professionalism have astonished me. It has given me great satisfaction to hand this method of treatment over to such a large number of homeopaths in the Netherlands. I feel sure that the rest of the world will follow.

Last but not least I want to thank, from the bottom of my heart, the hundreds of parents who have entrusted me with the healing of their son or daughter and who enabled me to gradually develop the CEASE therapy. Their feedback has guided me step by step to new possibilities and new hope for these children. A special word of thanks for the parents who in their testimonials have had the courage to tell the world what happened to their child.

Here I want to express also my compassion for all autistic and behaviorally-challenged children and their parents. I hope that in the near future all these parents and children will find the solution for their problem. Let us stop pretending that these children could change their behavior if they wanted to. Instead, let us understand that something is wrong with their brains which can be corrected with the method described in this book. In many ways it is our modern society that is responsible, and not the children. Realizing this will be a leap forward in the history of medical and psychological practice.

I am also extremely grateful for the Universal Intelligence that has created through me the CEASE therapy, as an effective tool to heal autistic as well as with other behavioral and neurological disorders.

Thanks finally to all those who have the courage to read this book and perhaps overcome some prejudices. Be inspired!

FOREWORD BY J.B. HANDLEY

I had the pleasure of meeting Tinus Smits at his office in the Netherlands and introducing him to my 5 year old son, Jamison, who was diagnosed with autism just before his second birthday.

Dr. Smits is an important voice in a new movement that has been growing by the day all over the world: parents, doctors and scientists who are helping children recover from autism and go on to lead the normal lives they were always meant to have.

One of the biggest challenges for doctors and parents alike involves choosing which treatment approach for autism to follow. Here in the United States, I'm aware of children who have recovered with diet, chelation, methyl B-12 injections, hyperbaric oxygen therapy, antiviral therapy, and homeopathy, to name just a few. How is a parent supposed to choose?

Dr. Smits' approach to treating autism, which this book covers in great detail, stands out among many others for its clarity, simplicity, and, perhaps most importantly, its focus on cause. The fact that it costs a fraction of some other therapies is a bonus and makes it accessible to parents staggering under the cost of treating their autistic child.

While Dr. Smits believes childhood vaccines administered before the age of two are a primary cause of autism, he explains how many of his patients also received other toxic insults (antibiotics, anesthesia, drugs, etc.) in their early years that contributed to autism. In addition, sometimes the cause turns out to be something the birth mother experienced before or during pregnancy.

By using Isotherapy -- the detoxification of toxic insults through homeo-pathic preparations -- Dr. Smits has found a novel way to approach two of autism's most complex challenges: reversing the comprehensive (and not yet fully understood) damage these toxic insults can cause to a child, and zeroing in on the toxins that affected each individual child.

With Isotherapy, you quickly learn which insults impacted which child, based on the reaction your child has to each preparation. In one child, Isotherapy with an MMR-derived homeopathic remedy may lead to healing while with another it may be detoxification from antibiotics or from a medicine a mother took while pregnant. Through his years of practice, Dr. Smits also draws on elements of classical homeopathy and naturopathy to tailor his approach to the needs of each individual child.

If you are an American picking up this book for the first time, homeopathy is probably a foreign concept to you. If you were raised in Europe, homeopathy is probably something you grew up using, understanding, and benefiting from. With more than 200 years of successful use, homeopathy is a well-practiced form of medicine that I believe is ideally suited for autism treatment: it's extremely safe, it's always individualized, it's comprehensive, and it respects that the human body knows best. Homeopathy gives each child's complex biology the chance to heal without suppressing the body's natural gift of healing.

If you are a practitioner treating children with autism or considering treating children with autism, I hope you will give this book a thorough and considered read. In Dr. Smits' limited practice with several hundred children, he has seen incredible results from his CEASE therapy.

With its safety, inexpensiveness, ease of use, and individualization, I hope many thousands more parents get the chance to experience first hand what so many of the parents working with Dr. Smits' have seen: the full realization of who their child was meant to be.

J.B. Handley

Co-Founder Generation Rescue - Jenny McCarthy's autism organization

Foreword by Hans Reijnen

As a consequence of the efforts of Tinus opening up new horizons, we have arrived at the point in the world of Complementary and Alternative Medicine (CAM) where our treatments are no longer the privilege of a small minority of 'enlightened' consumers of health care who have given preference over the decades to be treated by a homeopath or acupuncturist. Through the positive results of alternative practitioners over many years the CAM world has built up a small but solid position in the general health care of Holland. But at the same time these results were not so firmly established and visible to the general public that CAM could grow steadily throughout the years. More often it has felt like rowing against the current. But years of Tinus' careful observations in his own practice may have changed all this.

Tinus has succeeded in combining some of the most effective methods of treatment available in different forms of natural medicine in a way that the overall results have increased and are applicable to a broad spectrum of patients. This has led to astonishing results. His integrative manner of thinking and treating has become an example for different professional organizations practicing natural medicine. His integrative method of treatment arose from his broad knowledge of alternative medicine, his development of a kind of natural instinct during the intensive complementary treatment of patients with cancer (Non-Toxic Tumor Therapy), his thorough knowledge of and experience with homeopathy and his extended experience with ADHD and autistic children. Combining his experience and successful treatment of many patients suffering from all kinds of other diseases like allergies, chronic fatigue, degenerative diseases, depressions, emotional instability, etc., he improved, step by step, his practical conception of healing.

The integrated treatment of Tinus, which I have come to call 'Smitsian medicine', includes much more than just homeopathy. Because of its integrated character and remarkable effectiveness, his method deserves much greater attention. He is focusing his treatment now on autism because the results for this category of patients can be classified as spectacular. But his treatment is in my opinion (and personal experience) highly appropriate for patients with a vast range of chronic complaints.

Tinus directs his very precise interviewing technique combined with a great intuition at the gathering of all the information about the damaging elements (causes) in the patient's anamnesis. Then he resolves these causes step by step, using the causative factors as homeopathic remedies in different potencies to clear the symptoms or disease with which they are connected. This technique is called Isotherapy. Tinus himself speaks of the clearance of various 'imprints', a term which fits perfectly with the newly emerging approach of bioinformatics therapy.

Tinus is for me a role model because he is a real researcher, not in its pure scientific sense, but as a practical physician. He investigates everything that might contribute in a natural way to the healing of his patients and if it is found to be effective and efficient, it gets a place in his protocol of treatment. This approach in pilot studies where the number of patients is over 50 should be applied more often to help medical science to progress. He is passionate to reveal the deeper causations of our common Western diseases not neglecting the emotional and mental implications of every patient that is under his treatment.

Tinus is a genuine physician and a real holistic thinker, as much a psychologist as a physician. Once he get his teeth in a case he does not let go. He not only wants to heal, but considers it his sacred duty; whoever heals is right, says an old adage in the medical world. He knows that many of the diseases around us are unnecessary if the knowledge he has gathered would only be put into practice. His battle against ignorance sometimes resembles the battle of David against Goliath (notwithstanding the fact that at 6 foot 5, Tinus is not such a small guy). It is a daunting task to tackle the official and sacrosanct vaccination program. But tackle it he has and in doing so he has faced personal and professional jeopardy. Nevertheless, Tinus shows a great compassion for suffering human beings and dedicates himself selflessly to this noble goal. He has worked one month out of every year for the last 15 years on a homeopathic project in Nepal, teaching homeopathic health assistants and supervising homeopathic Nepali doctors.

He is also a talented teacher for many of his homeopathic colleagues all over the world. Tinus has high expectations of himself, but also of his colleagues. He has a strong Hahnemanian attitude, saying: make it like I do, but do it exactly like me, otherwise you will not get the same results. Perhaps this is exactly the quality you need to achieve what he has done, the ability to open up new horizons. He first did that for already existing homeopathic remedies like Carcinosinum, Cuprum metallicum, Saccharum off. and others. Later he developed a number of new homeopathic remedies like Carcinosinum cum Cuprum, Lac maternum and Vernix caseosa. And likewise he used this same tenacity with his systematic isopathic approach of the Post-Vaccination Syndrome, with the development of his Inspiring Homeopathy, with the integral and homeopathic treatment of cancer patients with Non-Toxic Tumor Therapy and last but not least by his successful engagement in the fast growing problem of autism.

His treatment protocol for autism can successfully be used by every homeopath with a good basic knowledge and experience of homeopathy. His therapy is practical and can be mastered easily during a five days intensive training. As a result of his publications and teachings, many homeopaths have broadened their therapeutic skills with orthomolecular treatments and food interventions, which can be successfully used along with homeopathy. Conversely, a growing number of naturopaths make the step to homeopathy to be able to treat their patients on a deeper energetic level. For some therapists this step to a more integral way of treatment, as Tinus has taught, can be a big leap, but it can improve enormously their healing potential. This gives energetic medicine a more solid position in primary health care and it enables the holistic therapist to reach the level of a specialist. At the same time the development of Complementary and Alternative Medicine (CAM) in the Netherlands and everywhere in the world gains credibility.

Tinus has a huge number of enthusiastic patients under his treatment, who have chosen energetic and holistic healing as their preferred medicine. In different scientific disciplines such as biophysics and bio-cybernetics the interconnection between matter, energy and information has already been demonstrated. (L. de Broglie (1892-1987) and C.F. von Weizsäcker (1912-2007)).

All life is vibration and every disturbance has its own frequency. The central idea is that every pathogenic organism, every heavy metal, every toxin or disease makes imprints in the energetic system of the organism, as Tinus shows clearly in this book. The chronic problems that many people suffer from, just ask for a deeper, integral healing from inside which has now become increasingly more available in alternative medicine.

Hans Reijnen, *homeopathic physician, the Netherlands*

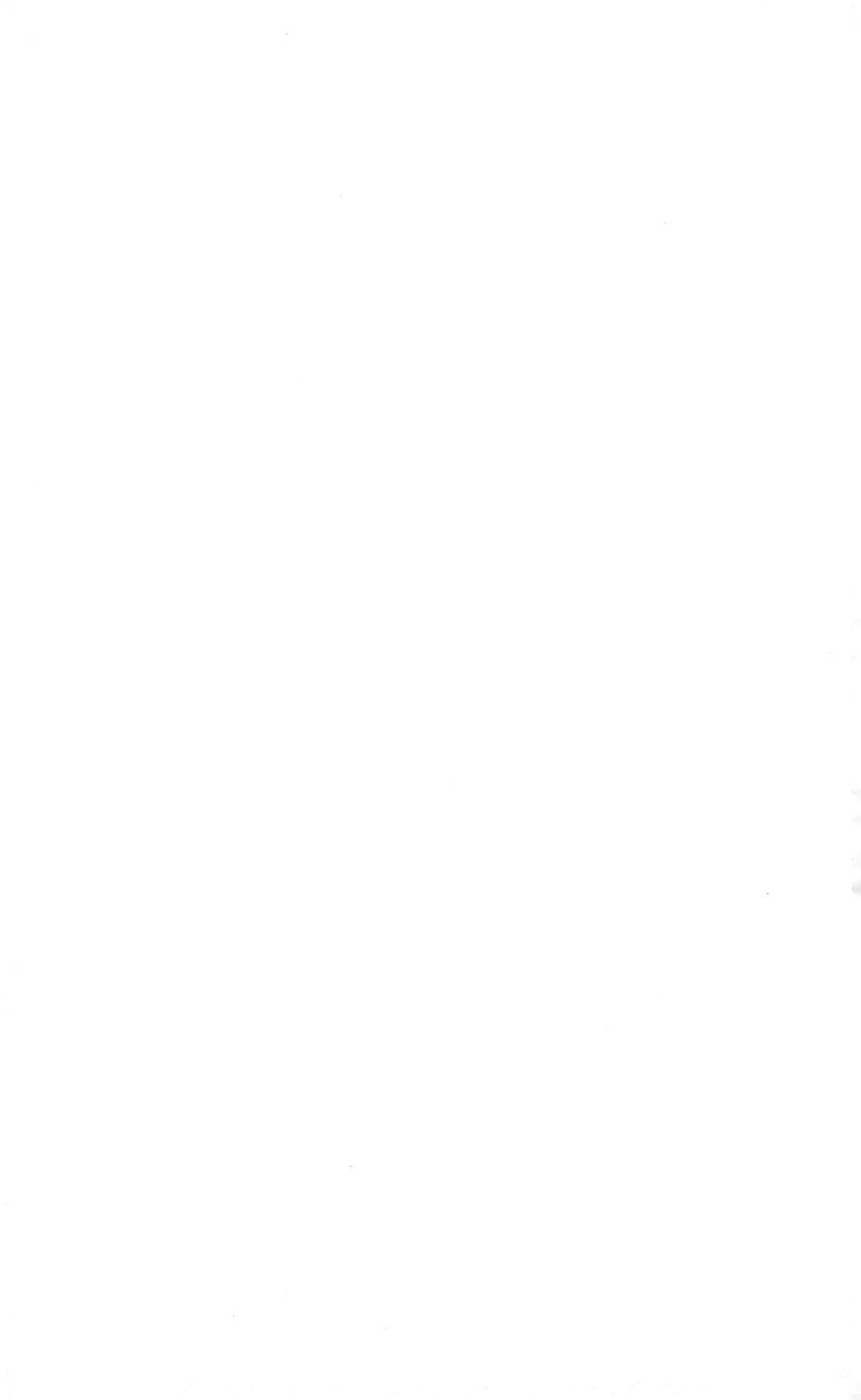

TABLE OF CONTENTS

CHAPTER 1

THE FIRST DISCOVERIES

My interest in autism was sparked by my experiences with detoxifying children who were damaged by vaccines. Many behavioral problems soon disappeared when vaccines were detoxified, even when many of these children came to me for completely different reasons. In my practice it turned out that mood swings, aggression, restlessness, attention deficit disorder (ADD) and ADHD were often correlated to the many and early vaccinations in children. When some of my autistic patients greatly improved after the detoxification of their vaccines, my interest was aroused, and I became increasingly convinced that autism must at least partially tie in with the administration of vaccines.

At a Chicago congress on autism in May of 2003 I presented 30 cases of behavioral disorders that had significantly improved with the detoxification of the vaccines (among these were three autistic children). Here I learned the latest scientific research on autism and became inspired by the many therapeutic possibilities these new insights offered. This is a message of hope, and I no longer consider it appropriate to label autism an incurable disorder. The facts simply disprove this assumption.

Over the last few years I have focused more and more on the treatment of these children and after having seen over 300 of them, regardless of what their diagnosis was or what the severity was, I came to the conclusion that by my treatment virtually every child can be considerably improved, even up to complete healing. I have named the treatment CEASE Therapy (Complete Elimination of Autistic Spectrum Expression). I say 'virtually all' because there are a few exceptions. When the cause of the deeper disturbance is not found, often because of a lack of information, then complete healing may not happen. Cure may not occur in cases with real brain damage as in certain brain diseases, in cases of strong epileptic fits or in post-meningitis or encephalitis cases.

But most autistic children are curable because their brains are not damaged but blocked. My journey through 300 cases of autism has been an exciting experience yielding the discovery of many causative factors. To guarantee the effectiveness of this CEASE therapy all over the world, I have decided to provide high-level training for certified homeopathic practitioners all over the world. In the coming years these methods may not yet be available in all countries, but our team will do its very best to make this wonderful treatment available at a very high standard to stop the suffering of these children and their families as soon as possible. In the Netherlands, homeopaths' interest in the first certification course was already overwhelming, with 85 homeopaths completing the course.

During the development of this treatment I became more and more aware that Isotherapy (i.e., using homeopathic preparations of the toxic substances that have caused the disease) gave me the key to wonderful healing processes. It also became clear to me that autism does not result from one single cause but rather from an accumulation of different causes. *So far the main obstacle to cure seems to be the lack of information about the causative factors. When important events in the life story of these children and their parents are overlooked or unknown, an essential key to the healing can be missed. When we know the causative factors in a child's life, we can almost always undo them with homeopathy.* This concept will become clear through case examples later in the book, such as the case in Chapter Three.

During my research for complete healing I became more and more amazed at how certain substances, even those not labeled as toxic, could be causative factors for autism or other developmental disorders.

For example, I saw a dramatic improvement in an autistic girl by the detox of a nasal spray, xylometazolin, which the mother had used regularly during her pregnancy. Conventional medicine (so often uses fundamentally toxic chemical substances) has become more and more of a pathogenic medicine. This is not only true for vaccines, but also for all kinds of treatments prescribed by my fellow doctors. When we prepare and use these same toxic substances as homeopathic remedies (more properly known as isopathic remedies), the profound toxic effects of these substances can be reversed and clearly linked to the patient's symptoms. You will find many examples in this book. The reactions to a needed isopathic remedy are so characteristic that the link between the causes and the effects are undeniable. In this way I discovered step by step why autism and other behavioral problems with specific developmental links have so dramatically increased over the last ten to twenty years with the increase in vaccines and prescription drugs for children.

With this isopathic treatment I also use orthomolecular medicine (nutritional supplements in therapeutic doses) to nourish the brains of these children and to restore proper intestinal function. Many supplements have some usefulness for the treatment of autism, but I have found only a few to be necessary, like Vitamin C, magnesium, zinc and fish oil. In my treatment these supplements serve as a support for the healing process which is actually being carried out by the isopathic treatment. These supplements make the whole healing process smoother and help minimize reactions to the detoxification. But it should be clearly noted that in my experience it is impossible to heal autism with supplements alone, simply because autism is not caused by the deficiency of certain vitamins or minerals. Nevertheless, with these supplements we regularly see steady improvements in the conditions of these children.

As a third arrow in my quiver, I also use classical homeopathy and Inspiring Homeopathy, which will be defined and discussed extensively in the next chapters. They both can play an important role in the complete healing of autistic children, although without the resolution of specific causes which are responsible for the development of autism, classical homeopathy alone rarely brings about complete healing. Nevertheless this way of healing can give very encouraging results as will be shown in this book. It must be said here clearly that this CEASE therapy can only be executed by well trained homeopathic practitioners.

In this book many new concepts will be introduced as part of a system of healing which is so radically different from conventional medicine that it is difficult to believe and difficult to assimilate. These new concepts will become increasingly clear with the many case examples provided. I suggest that readers new to homeopathy read the entire book at least twice and refer to the glossary at the end for unfamiliar terms. The CEASE therapy will be much more believable and understandable the second time around.

If we fail to take the right measures, a continuously and rapidly growing number of our children will become severely handicapped in the near future. A much greater awareness is also necessary concerning the use of medical drugs during pregnancy and delivery. Every chemical substance that is unnatural is potentially toxic. The statement that drugs are safe for use during pregnancy just tells the doctor that there are no *known* genetic disturbances or major side-effects, but that does not mean that they are safe. Sometimes doctors have no choice, as in epilepsy, colitis, malignant hypertension, asthma, emergency surgery, etc. But many of the inconveniences of pregnancy like acid reflux, morning sickness, premature contractions, etc. can be cured easily with natural medicine and homeopathy. Parents should choose the non-toxic option first and be aware of the possible side-effects of regular drugs for the unborn baby. Also food and drinks should be an issue of importance for the future mother. Organic food should be the preference. With the CEASE therapy we are now investigating glutamates, aspartame, and plastic softeners as possible causative factors for autism.

With the creation of the CEASE Therapy and the CEASE Organization, it is my dream that this treatment will become readily available all over the world. In this way parents can choose if and how they want their child to be healed, because *healing is possible*. Let us stop calling autism an incurable disease; the facts simply contradict this view. In the near future we can begin research to document the effectiveness of this approach.

CHAPTER 2

HOMEOPATHY HAS THE ANSWERS

Different types of homeopathy and their healing potential
To understand fully the potential of homeopathy, we have to consider which type of homeopathy can achieve our goal of completely healing autism. In other disease conditions, the most elegant and powerful way to heal a patient is with classical homeopathy (using a single remedy to cover the totality of mental, emotional, and physical symptoms), which will be discussed later in this chapter. But in my experience classical homeopathy alone is rarely sufficient to achieve complete healing in autism, although it can sometimes give very significant improvement. The key to the healing of autism with homeopathy is not the classical homeopathic approach but Isotherapy (using a homeopathic remedy made from a safe preparation of the toxic causative agent), as you will learn throughout this book.

Pathways of transfer from mother to child
The health of our children begins with the health of both father and mother before conception. Then many factors, both prenatal and in early childhood, affect the overall health of the child: medication, vaccination, food, environmental intoxication (poisoning); the use of drugs during pregnancy; the quality of the pregnancy itself; the delivery (with or without medication); the medical history; and especially the use of drugs on the child during the first two years of the life. Pregnancy and early childhood are decisive for the later health status of our children.

The brain of an unborn baby and of a baby under the age of two is extremely sensitive to all kinds of influences and can easily be harmed by chemical substances. Fat-soluble molecules, including those of oxygen and carbon dioxide, anesthetics, and alcohol can pass straight through the lipids in the capillary walls and so gain access to all parts of the brain. Especially in the first three months of the fetus the blood-brain barrier is not fully formed, Sometimes these substances cannot be avoided. For that reason parents and doctors should be extremely careful with the administration of any substance that is unnatural or chemical. Any drug, even one considered safe for the unborn child, should be considered as potentially toxic, based on my experience in having to counteract the effects of these drugs. Later in this book you will find many cases where medication during pregnancy has contributed substantially to the development of autism or other behavioral problems. Sometimes drugs or diseases even from before the pregnancy can play an important role and have to be corrected with homeopathy.

To understand fully how the health of our future children is affected, it is important to know that their health during the pregnancy and the first two years depends on three different means of transmission from the mother to the child:

Genetic transfer: as we know, the child receives half of its genes from each parent. It has to be said that most children are born genetically healthy. Autism is often referred to as a genetic disease, but a genetic disease cannot increase within one generation as rapidly as autism has.

Material transfer: toxins can pass through the umbilical cord during pregnancy, including heavy metals, drugs the mother takes, alcohol, tobacco, toxic products in her food, etc. Once the baby is born, toxins can enter via its food (breast feeding or bottle feeding), by the air it is inhaling (for example from fresh paint and vinyl covering on the floor of a baby's bedroom), through its still very permeable skin (shampoo, soap and creams with parabens, ethyl glycol, phthalates, bisphenol A, etc.) and by medication (antibiotics, anesthesia, vaccines, etc.).

Energetic transfer: this form of transmission needs special explanation because it is hardly known or even acknowledged in the medical world, but plays a crucial role in understanding how our children are damaged and become autistic or have other behavioral or developmental problems. Substances that are toxic can damage the unborn or young baby not only by their material toxicity but also by creating an imprint in the baby's energetic field, its vital energy. Diseases can do the same. Toxic substances cause acute reactions when the material concentration of the toxin is at its highest. When this concentration diminishes, the toxic effects decrease and finally disappear completely. But the toxic substance can leave an energetic imprint that lasts even after the material substance is no longer present, especially after longterm exposure to the toxin. This explains why chelation therapy is often not enough to heal the toxicity induced by heavy metal poisoning. Generally, toxins can have lifelong effects if irreparable tissue damage has taken place or if the toxin has provoked an energetic imprint in the energetic system (vital energy) of the patient.

Recently I came across an interesting article in a French magazine *Nexus*, July-August 2009, no.63, page 82-88, mentioning the research of Nora Bénachour and Gilles-Eric Séralini from the University of Caen published in *Chemical Research in Toxicology*, December 2008. They studied the toxicology of high dilutions of the pesticide Roundup produced by Monsanto. They came to the conclusion that concentrations 100,000 times lower than that to which a normal gardener is exposed still kills cells in newborns. This shows again how careful we have to be with toxins during pregnancy and the first years of life. This conception of energetic imprints explains the success of homeopathic treatments, especially of Isotherapy, which directly targets these toxic imprints. I do not know of any other therapy that is able to reverse this energetic damage effectively. Done well, this isopathic treatment enables the homeopath to guide the patient to complete healing. Before going more deeply into the realm of Isotherapy, let us first have a look at another important aspect of homeopathic treatment to understand why we use different potencies.

Use of different potencies

Dr. Samuel Hahnemann, the founder of homeopathy, pioneered the use of remedies in different potencies (strengths), derived by a process called serial dilution and succussion. The more times a substance has been diluted and succussed (energized), the higher the potency and the more powerful and deep working the action. Remedies are labeled according to their potency with 30C being a relatively low potency, 200C being a medium potency, and 1M (C1000) or 10M (C10,000) being high potencies.

Hahnemann noticed that if a certain potency had finished its healing action and the disease was not yet completely erased, a higher potency was often necessary to continue the healing process. Thus, a remedy is often used in an ascending sequence (typically in my practice 30C, 200C, 1M and 10M, sometimes up to the 50M potency) to clear out an energetic disturbance. When we use Isotherapy, different levels of energetic disturbance or disease are often brought clearly forward. When a patient has finished the detoxification from the 30C potency and is no longer reacting to it, that does not mean that the detoxification is complete. As soon as the next potency (200C) is given, a clear reaction is once again possible. Some children react to all the potencies, others only to one or two potencies.

The conclusion we can draw from these experiences is that a disease (i.e., an energetic disturbance) can occur within a narrow energetic range or over a broad range. In general, we can say that low potencies are more active on the physical plane, while the higher potencies are effective for more emotional and mental issues. To clear the whole range of different energetic levels, I use as a basic treatment for every detoxification the 30C, 200C, 1M and 10M potencies (which I refer to as 'a course' of the remedy).

Trauma-related and constitutional (inborn) disturbances

To treat autism successfully, it is important to understand the difference between disturbances created by a specific trauma and those that are part of the inborn nature of the patient, addressed by what is called 'constitutional' homeopathy. These two types of disturbances will need different types of treatment, so it is important to distinguish them.

A trauma-related disturbance can be attributed to a specific toxic exposure or event that has left an imprint in the patient's energy field. This can be a vaccine, a food additive, an environmental toxin, or a drug used during the pregnancy or the first two years of life. It can also be an important emotional trauma, like the death of another child while the mother is pregnant, or a hospitalization early in life. In fact, homeopaths always choose remedies based on this kind of cause when it exists, not just on the effects (symptoms), except in life-threatening circumstances. Professional homeopaths always look for causations in their patients and choose a remedy that can eliminate the disturbing energy and restore the patient's energetic balance. When the cause is emotional, it will become part of the choice of a constitutional remedy in classical homeopathy. When it is a toxin, it can be better addressed by a targeted remedy made from that specific substance which does not attempt to address the entire mental-emotional makeup of the patient. Using this type of toxin-based remedy to heal a specific physical disturbance is what we call Isotherapy.

The constitutional treatment of a patient applies a different principle of homeopathic medicine. The constitution of a patient can be defined as the combination of deep disturbances throughout life and generations of family histories that have influenced the patient's life energy. There are not a specific number of clear disturbances, as in autism, but a unique and distinctive energetic pattern that matches a specific homeopathic remedy, derived from a plant, animal or mineral source. It is the task of a classical homeopath to discover the homeopathic remedy which resonates most closely with the character and peculiar symptoms that the patient shows us. This well chosen remedy is called the *simillimum*, the remedy that fits the patient's energetic pattern completely at a very deep level and which is able to initiate a deep healing process at the physical, emotional, mental and even spiritual level. Such a constitutional remedy is based on the whole energy pattern and does not cover just a specific disturbance as does Isotherapy.

Many homeopaths still believe that everything can be healed by classical homeopathy (constitutional treatment). But in my experience, classical homeopathy alone is not enough to cure autism. So in my method of treatment, it is of the first importance for the treating homeopath to see where to apply constitutional homeopathy and to proceed step by step to heal the specific causes of disease with Isotherapy.

Isotherapy

Isotherapy, as previously noted, is the use of pathogenic products in homeopathic potencies. When a certain substance is suspected to have contributed to the development of autism, this substance can be given in homeopathic potencies. For example, in a case where the MMR vaccination is suspected, we prescribe a course of homeopathic MMR in 30C, 200C, 1M and 10M potencies to remove the possible imprint that the MMR vaccine has left, especially in the brain. Because, in my experience, autism is caused by an accumulation of different toxins and traumas, its treatment with Isotherapy consists of the use of a number of different potentized substances. For example, the treatment of an autistic child over a certain period of time can be as follows: detoxification of the MMR, NeisVac-C (meningococcus), DTPP/Hib, and Fenoterol (a drug used to delay premature labor). This brings the child step by step to the complete elimination of these disturbing imprints, with tremendous improvement of all autistic features.

The reactions to these treatments are quite often very significant: the child may once again experience the same symptoms it had when first given the vaccination or other drug. For example, in the detoxification of a vaccine the parents report that the child again has the 'brain cry', or is sleepy for days or is angry and irritable, just like in the days after that particular vaccination. Physical detoxification as a reaction to this isopathic treatment is also very common: runny nose, ears and/ or eyes; diarrhea, sweating, skin eruptions and fever. This is where the anti-oxidants I recommend (vitamin C, zinc, magnesium, ascorbyl palmitate and fish oil) are especially useful in preventing overly strong detox reactions and to support the physical condition of the child.

In fact, the use of Isotherapy gives us valuable information as to what symptoms were provoked by what causation. With Isotherapy the toxic effects of vaccinations can no longer be denied. But Isotherapy also teaches us that vaccinations are not the only cause of autism, nor are mercury or aluminum the only harmful substances in the shots. As mentioned earlier in this text even an 'innocent' nasal spray used by the mother during pregnancy can contribute greatly to the development of autism.

Isotherapy also allows us to determine whether certain suspected events in the medical or life history of the patient are causative factors. If there is no reaction to the detoxification of a certain substance, we can conclude that this substance had nothing to do with the child's autism. If, on the contrary, there are clear reactions to the homeopathic preparation of a suspected substance followed by clear improvements, we can just as readily conclude that the original substance was harmful.

We also have the means to verify whether a given detoxification has been complete or not. When we see clear reactions to a given course of a remedy and we repeat it several times only to find no reaction to the last repetition of the course, we can reasonably conclude that the detoxification of that substance has been successfully completed and the next step can be taken. This usually happens after a potency has been given in repeated doses as long as reactions take place, followed by a last complete repetition of the whole course to verify nothing is left. Finally, it means that all the information of a toxic substance or disease has been completely removed from the patient's energy field.

With all these causative factors to remove, Isotherapy is the main tool in the successful treatment of autism. Nevertheless, for full healing it can be necessary to also use other forms of homeopathy like Inspiring Homeopathy and classical homeopathy to heal the innate health problems (constitution) not caused by the specific causations that have to be resolved by Isotherapy.

Inspiring Homeopathy

Inspiring Homeopathy is a modern form of classical homeopathy I developed to treat universal human problems, which I have labeled universal layers. The focus of Inspiring Homeopathy is on the life processes of the patient. The themes I have so far uncovered are *want of self-confidence, lack of (self)love, lack of incarnation (grounding in the body), lack of protection, old traumas, guilt, and disconnection from the Self.*

Inspiring Homeopathy can help the patient to become aware that he is spiraling around the same problem or issue, continuously repeating the same experiences. It catalyzes the resolution of deeper problems and helps the person to become more himself. Not only can it help the patient with life issues and self-awareness, Inspiring Homeopathy has proved to play an important role in modern diseases such as cancer, ADHD, aggressive behavior and autism. The most frequently prescribed remedies for these layers in autism are Cuprum metallicum, which can very nicely heal the obsessiveness, inflexibility and tension including tics and head banging, and Saccharum officinale, which has a wonderful action on the affective part of the problem, restoring emotional contact with parents, siblings and classmates. Saccharum can help these kids to understand what others feel and help them to express once again their own feelings. Sometimes other remedies used in Inspiring Homeopathy can help as well, for example to create better boundaries against external stimuli (Vernix caseosa), to be more present and grounded in their body (Lac maternum) or to heal their aggressiveness (Anacardium orientale).

Nevertheless these remedies cannot replace the treatment with Isotherapy. If the fundamental imbalance is not corrected with the right isotherapeutic remedy, Inspiring or classical homeopathic remedies can usually only heal to a certain extent. In the next chapter Inspiring Homeopathy will be explored more extensively with case examples because this form of homeopathy is still relatively unknown by the general public and even by homeopathic practitioners.

Classical Homeopathy

Classical homeopathy, the original homeopathy invented and developed by Dr. Samuel Hahnemann 200 years ago, is still the predominant approach used by homeopaths worldwide. All the different variations developed later. The basic principles of homeopathy are all derived from the classical approach: find the unique remedy (the similimum) at the deepest level of the patient and use it to provoke resonance in the patient and thereby restore his lost equilibrium. There are thousands of remedies derived from plant, mineral, chemical, animal and human sources. The process requires a broad professional knowledge: a deep insight into human functioning, an extended knowledge of the remedies and their classification (materia medica) and sufficient experience. When a remedy has been well chosen it leads to wonderful healing processes. In my experience this form of homeopathy is generally not the most appropriate for the resolution of the disturbances called autism, that should preferably be corrected with the right isotherapeutic remedy. If classical homeopathy had been effective on a large scale in the treatment of autism, this form of homeopathy would already be established as a first choice approach for autism; this is far from the case.

Clinical Homeopathy and complex homeopathy

Instead of prescribing a remedy based on the totality of the symptoms as in classical homeopathy, clinical homeopathy focuses only on a certain disease or organ. Lower potencies are usually the most effective for this type of physical problems. They can be repeated every day or even two or three times a day. That is why I use a D6 (low potency) of Saccharum officinale once a day to heal the digestive system of autistic children with great success. In the same way Chelidonium and Cholesterinum can be used to detoxify the liver and Berberis to stimulate the kidneys. When organs are detoxified and stimulated, this is called drainage therapy.

Some homeopaths reject this kind of homeopathy as a misapplication of the healing principles developed by Dr. Hahnemann. In my opinion, we have to use all the possibilities that this wonderful way of healing offers us. Isotherapy, clinical homeopathy and classical homeopathy can be combined effectively and lead to more successful treatment.

When several remedies of clinical use are combined in one formula, it becomes complex homeopathy. I do not use these combined formulas, but I sometimes prescribe several clinical remedies at the same time, especially in cancer therapy, where the liver, the digestive system, and the kidneys are often severely burdened during chemo or radiation therapy. Many of these combination remedies are sold over the counter as self help products and deserve their place there.

Nosode Therapy

Nosode therapy has much in common with Isotherapy, because it uses homeopathic remedies made from a disease-causing microbe or diseased tissue (of course safely diluted so that no trace of the original substance remains). Remedies such as Syphilinum, Carcinosinum, Tuberculinum, Mononucleosis, Borrelia (Lyme disease nosode) and many others are frequently used even in classical homeopathy. Nosode therapy is a very direct method for removing the imprints that a disease has left in the energetic body of the patient. Patients often complain that they have never completely recovered after a particular disease. The administration of the nosode for that disease can completely resolve such disturbance and restore the state of health as it existed before the disease.

Organ therapy

To stimulate specific organ systems, homeopathic remedies made from the same organ can be used (with the actual tissue taken from the organs of sheep, calf or pig). Such therapy is especially useful when an organ is damaged or functioning at a low energy level, usually at the same time as deeper homeopathic treatment. In a C4 or C5 potency these organ remedies have a stimulating action and can greatly help in the recovery of a specific organ or area. I have seen e.g. nice results in cancer patients with severe anemia or leucopenia (too low white blood cells) because of chemotherapy, which often suppresses the production of blood cells in the bone marrow. Medulla ossium (a homeopathic preparation of bone marrow) C4, 10 drops twice a day greatly stimulates the manufacture of red and white blood cells and eliminates the anemia or leucopenia. Even given preventively during chemotherapy it works nicely.

CHAPTER 3

THE MULTIFACTORIAL TREATMENT

As a homeopathic physician, I now possess different ways to bring suffering children out of their isolation and restore them to an interactive and emotional world. To be more specific, the treatments I use include:

1. The detoxification of the various vaccines and other causative factors using homeopathically prepared remedies made from these factors that possibly triggered the autism.

2. The supplemental administration of omega-3 fatty acids (fish oil with EPA and DHA) to restore the integrity of the brain functions.

3. The use of relatively high doses of Vitamin C (both water and fat soluble).

4. The homeopathic treatment of the child with Inspiring Homeopathy and classical homeopathy to treat the disturbances that are not directly linked with toxic substances but with constitutional disturbances.

5. Orthomolecular treatment to restore the copper/zinc ratio and to reactivate the metallothionein. The heavy metal level will thereby be decreased gradually and the integrity of the intestines restored. I usually administer zinc and magnesium as part of a complex with vitamin C to reduce the number of pills the child has to take daily. For dosages see chapter 12.

6. The use of healthy, organic food without sugar and other additives, and the use of Saccharum officinale in a D6 potency, one tablet every day, to restore the integrity of the intestines. Saccharum is a wonderful remedy for the digestive system in general and can heal the insatiable appetite many autistic children have.

Different theories

It has often been shown that autistic children can benefit greatly from classical homeopathic treatment, whether physically or emotionally. Yet it is my experience that there is still room for improvement if we acquire a deeper understanding of the autistic state. Many theories have been presented as to the cause of autism. One theory claims autism to be a genetic disorder and for that reason considers it incurable. Certainly, within the medical world, this is probably the most widespread and persistent conviction. Likewise, there are some 'alternative' views. Autistic children are said to be unwilling or unable to incarnate. Sometimes these children are seen as 'new age' children who have come into this world with a special mission in order to help us. Others claim that a 'wrong' part of these children has incarnated and therefore it is impossible for them to participate in this world. There are many adherents to the theory that autism is caused by heavy metals and chelating therapy is advised. The theory that mercury in vaccines is the main culprit is widespread especially in the United States. Again others claim that these children lack certain enzymes or have a problem with methylation, which can be resolved respectively by cod liver oil and methyl cobalamin. Others are not focusing on causations but try to improve the behavior and functioning of autistic children with behavioral therapy, Sonrise and ABA being the most important forms.

In my experience, autism has multiple causations, primarily toxins but also inherited energetic patterns from the parents. This approach will be explained further in the next chapter, but first let us look at a case which illustrates this multifactorial approach.

An instructive case of multiple causations and a multifactorial treatment

From some cases we can learn a lot; both the problems confronted and their cure give us insight into the underlying disturbances and how these problems can be solved. Here two homeopathic remedies, Saccharum officinale and Cuprum metallicum, worked wonderfully. The case of Bjorn gave me a great deal of insight into the functioning of autistic children. By age ten he had not been formally diagnosed as autistic, but he had had severe behavioral problems dating back eight and a half years. Over the course of eight years his parents went from one institution to another, from the pediatrician to the psychiatrist, to the psychologist, to the social worker and to the counselor. Many thick reports were written and numerous tests performed. The mother stated that the help she had gotten so far was miserable. When I saw Bjorn the situation at school was intolerable, but nobody knew where to put him. The director of the school said he had never seen such wretched behavior.

Underlying disturbances leading to severe behavior problems

It all started suddenly at a year and a half, one week before the birth of his brother. Bjorn would scream virtually the entire day over a period of two and a half years, driving his parents mad. He became defiant, not accepting any limitations. Emotionally, there was no progress during these years. He seemed not to be touched by anything. He functioned completely on his mental skills, inventing the most horrible torments for his parents or coach. He would look straight into your eyes to sense in what way you were affected by his tricks. He had a special knack for choosing his victims. He could hardly be tested because there was no cooperation. The most precise diagnosis was: 'Maybe some kind of autistic spectrum disturbance, maybe PDD-NOS

(Pervasive Developmental Disorder, not otherwise specified – basically a catchall diagnosis when doctors cannot be more specific).' There was a lot of acting-out behavior. Sometimes he showed a completely different side and could be very sensitive and concerned. He needed a very strict approach without much space for his excesses. He had almost no contact with other children.

During the pregnancy his mother was given antibiotics twice for skin problems. The delivery was 'very problematic'; the labor was induced. Spinal anesthesia was attempted three times but failed. The amniotic fluid contained meconium and Bjorn was born with the umbilical cord around his neck. As a baby he was quiet. He got his bottle after it was warmed up in the microwave. He received his vaccinations without much trouble. At nine months his mother fell down the stairs with her baby in her arms. His skull got a little crack, which was not treated. At age four he had varicella (chickenpox).

He complained frequently about headaches, but a scan did not reveal anything. He also complained frequently about pain in his abdomen (both problems can be treated homeopathically with Saccharum officinale). His speech developed quite late, around age three and even then his speech developed too slowly. At four he was given speech therapy.

I tell his story in detail to show how all the events in a child's life, including those of the pregnancy, can contribute to the development of autism. Failure to understand these details can hide the key to the cure of his autism or whatever diagnosis could be put on it. Homeopathy offers wonderful tools to clear out the energetic imprints of these events by the homeopathic preparation of the substances that were responsible for them.

This boy's emotional and social skills were blocked. He was not able to show or feel compassion. In many autistic children we see the same thing. Because the vaccines were not directly suspected and there was no clear causation where we could focus the treatment, I decided to start first with Saccharum to stimulate his social/emotional skills. This remedy has proved to be able to restore in many cases the emotionality and social behavior lacking in autistic children. In addition to the Saccharum I prescribed Cuprum to heal his obsessive tendency to harm other people and to make him more flexible and adaptable. Cuprum is a wonderful remedy for making autistic children less obsessive, more flexible and relaxed and more capable of coping with stress. This combination of Saccharum and Cuprum has already helped many autistic children in their healing process. I gave both remedies once a week in a 30C potency, along with ascorbyl palmitate 500mg capsules, two of them three times a day, and ascorbate complex 1000mg tablets, one tablet three times a day. This complex also contains 82mg of potassium, 60mg of magnesium, 3mg of zinc and 75mg of bioflavonoids. Along with this I advised his parents not to use the microwave any more and to have Bjorn receive an osteopathic treatment for his head injury in infancy.

Three months later he was another child. After two weeks of treatment there was already a clear improvement. He started to sleep better and woke up cheerful in the morning. He was calmer, started to tell stories from school and was more open to social contacts. After school he left the house to find other children, first by putting small invitations on paper in the mailbox, later by ringing the doorbell and asking if the child wanted to play with him. He also started to write down his feelings. He became more and more independent. His abdominal pain disappeared completely and his headache was much better. His concentration also became much better. His extreme fear of dogs disappeared, and he even started to pet dogs he didn't know without any fear. He even allowed his brother to touch him, and he was able to play with him normally, where before every physical contact made him angry.

At school this big change did not go unobserved. He became much more socially adapted and could, for the most part, be kept in the classroom instead of outside. His acting-out behavior and tricks almost completely vanished. There was also the good news that he was accepted to stay at his school for the next year.

Saccharum and Cuprum together with the supplements were able to launch the healing process right away and remove the blockage he had on the social/emotional level. The treatment was continued with a higher potency (200C) of both the homeopathic remedies.

Half a year later his behavior was still excellent. He had grown enormously in approachability and independence. At school he was performing at the highest level and his concentration was very good. His headache and abdominal pains had almost completely gone. The only problem that still worried the parents and the school was his lack of social skills. He often sought negative attention or withdrew completely from the group.

With my growing experience over the last years I have learned that these classical remedies usually cannot bring the patient to complete healing because the energetic imprints of vaccines and of other drugs or events have to be resolved with Isotherapy first. Although it is tempting to look for the next single remedy that can heal the remaining symptoms (as in classical homeopathy or Inspiring Homeopathy), many of these cases get stuck because the specific detoxification with Isotherapy is not properly understood.

At this point of his treatment I decided to detoxify his vaccinations starting with the NeisVac-C over four weeks, then the MMR and finally the DTPP/Hib. On the NeisVac-C detoxification an enormous cleansing process took place. He had a long lasting diarrhea and headache. It took five months to give the whole course twice; the control course lasted only one month because there were no reactions anymore. That meant that this vaccine had been properly treated and would not affect his system any longer. The improvement on this course was not so evident: he played more with his brother, which was new, but with other children he could suddenly interrupt the play and refuse to play further. His overall behavior stayed acceptable and his intentions were good. Then the MMR and DTPP/Hib were detoxified with much milder reactions than on the Neisvac-C, but his behavior at home and at school improved considerably during the months after the clearance of these two vaccines. He was more involved, although he remained socially awkward. He pushed the limits of other children and did not function well among his peers. He also had obsessive thoughts, which made him nervous, especially in the evening in bed. It was clear that all the causations had not yet been resolved in this child.

At this point I presented my checklist to the parents. This checklist has proved to be very effective and has already revealed many causations which stayed hidden before. This checklist gave very valuable information about how to continue Bjorn's treatment. During the pregnancy his mother had skin infections for which she was given several courses of antibiotics, and she used aspartame in her coffee to avoid to putting on too much weight. She incidentally used the nasal spray xylomethazolin, plus Bjorn was also given this nose spray during his frequent colds. He was bottle fed from birth, and his mother put the plastic bottle in the microwave to warm his milk. She did this for about two years.

All this information gathered with the checklist gives good indications to continue his treatment and to try to get complete healing. So I have prescribed for Bjorn a homeopathic remedy made from plastic softeners which have been warmed up in the microwave, a remedy produced by the Hahnemann pharmacy in Holland. Next will be a remedy made from xylomethazolin, then homeopathic aspartame, and finally a remedy made from a mixture of antibiotics (Poli-antibioticum).

This treatment is still underway as of this writing. Updates of his treatment will be posted on my website www.cease-autism.com when the results of these four treatments will be known. But already this case is a beautiful example of our procedure. When I ask the parents how far we are in the overall healing of Bjorn they answer at least 60%, a nice result so far.

You will find many cases further on in this book, which show the healing power of Isotherapy. In this case I just wanted to show some practical applications of Inspiring Homeopathy and the detoxification with Isotherapy. It is my strong conviction that all children with behavioral problems should be treated by experienced homeopaths before they become adolescents and wind up in special boarding schools or even in jail. Homeopathy gives us the possibility to heal the brain and to bring these children back to normal social and emotional functioning. They deserve better than a repressive and authoritarian approach, which has proven for centuries not to be effective. In Chapter 9 on aggressiveness you will find extensive information with cases about this subject.

CHAPTER 4

THE GENESIS OF AUTISM

Through analyzing the healing processes of more than 300 autistic children, I came to a personal vision of how autism can be explained and treated. It would be of little value if this working hypothesis did not fit perfectly with all these wonderful healings that have been achieved by gradually developing an effective protocol. Little by little it became evident which information should be collected and what should be treated with priority.

To be sure, the scientific confirmation of this working hypothesis is not within easy reach because multi-causal approaches are difficult to test. Fortunately all the millions of autistic children worldwide do not have to wait for scientific confirmation before beginning the protocol. They and their parents are just interested in the healing itself and their success will be a testimonial for other parents and children. And in fact, an analysis of my cases has been started already and a pilot study will be started in 2010 with a few autistic children to prepare for a larger research project to study the effectiveness of the CEASE therapy.

My initial approach resulted from my decades-long experience with healing many behavioral and other problems in children through the detoxification of vaccines. As a result of this success, I wondered if it was correct to accuse the multi vaccination program for the enormous increase of these diseases. Certainly, over the last ten years there has been a groundswell of many parents, doctors, scientists and children's organizations becoming increasingly critical about the side-effects of vaccines. But I wondered about how to prove whether they were right or wrong. How can we prove that a certain event or medication is causative for the development of autism?

I came to believe that there are some substances apparently so toxic to the brain that they are capable of completely disturbing its normal functioning, especially from conception up to the age of two years. I also came to understand that not every substance that is unhealthy for human beings or babies is responsible for the development of autism, e.g., sugar and other sweets and refined food. Unhealthy does not necessarily mean causative.

Because most children are born healthy and have an initial normal development, how do we account for a child who suddenly regress and loses the capabilities that he had already developed in the first 12 to 24 months? What makes the difference between a child that continues to grow up in a healthy and prosperous way and a child that suddenly stops thriving and even regresses. Is there one specific toxic substance or is it a combination of many? Is there something in our environment that we still have not identified and that attacks the brains of children with weak immune systems, since we see so many autistic children with chronic runny noses, ear infections, bronchitis, digestive problems, etc., all signs of a weakened immune system? Is autism really curable or is it an incurable disease as so many doctors and even researchers believe?

And if we claim a genetic disorder is responsible, how is it possible then that autism has increased by more than 100%, even 150% in the last few years, while a genetic disease can increase only 3 to 4% in one generation (30 years). And how do we explain the many healings all over the world if genetics is the main reason? No, the genetic theory as the main causative factor cannot hold. Genetics can give a certain predisposition, but not more than that. Finally, is autism a preventable disease and if so, how? Many, many questions remained unanswered in my mind, some have been resolved, others not.

I am not a scientist but just a homeopathic doctor who wants to heal these little creatures who suddenly become wrecks instead of a joy for their parents. After seeing all this suffering, I decided to find out if autistic children really can heal 100%. Yes, 100%, not just 50% or 75%. To identify all the causes that have generated this enormous breakdown in our children, I felt that I had to reach the point of complete healing to be sure that I had uncovered everything that contributes to the development of autism. By implication if all the causative factors were detected then it would be possible that any autistic child could be healed. In other words, the eradication of all causative factors in a child should automatically lead to complete healing.

Or have these supposed toxins caused real damage to the brain tissue that is impossible to heal anymore? At the time I embarked on this project, this last theory was already contradicted by my experiences with the detoxification of all kinds of behavioral problems in non-autistic children and in some autistic children as well. True, I had not yet arrived at complete healing with the majority of autistic children, but had already reached a range of 50 to 80%.

But, I wondered, do we necessarily have to treat them at a very young age; is it too late for older children and adults? I had so many questions that I felt could only be answered by clinical experience.

Over the last three years working with about 300 autistic children, I have discovered with the help of Isotherapy which factors are involved in the genesis of autism and many other childhood disturbances. Many of the above questions can now be answered:

- Yes, all autistic children can be healed!

- No, autism is not just a vaccination problem or a heavy metal problem, or a leaky gut syndrome.

- No, there is not just one reason for autism; autism is an accumulation of different causative factors.

- Yes, autism can be healed during adolescence and even during adulthood.

- No, autism is not just provoked by factors in the first or second year of the child's lifetime.

- Yes, pregnancy and even the period before pregnancy can play a decisive role.

As a homeopathic physician I have a wonderful tool at my disposal: Isotherapy. I have already had extensive experience with it and know how to handle the detoxification of all kinds of toxins. I have healed many children and adults using the homeopathic preparation of all kinds of substances that had caused damage to the energetic system.

It is my belief and experience that the genetic theory which claims that autism is incurable is untenable. A child's genetics can only contribute to a certain vulnerability to contracting autism through a variety of injuries to healthy brain function. But autism is not the result of permanent damage to the brain tissue; it is just a blockage which makes proper brain performance impossible. Autism is not a permanent physical disease but an energetic disease.

That is why Isotherapy is the perfect tool to bring these children back. Yes, there is some weakness in autistic children, and, not surprisingly, one of the side-effects of this isotherapeutic treatment is the empowerment of the immune system and the disappearance of chronic runny noses, repeated ear infections, bronchitis, throat infections, GI infections, etc. Yes, autism is a preventable disease in most cases.

If everybody understood how a little child can become autistic, many preventive measures could be taken to dramatically reduce the number of autistic children all over the world. To this end we should counsel parents to prepare well before the pregnancy; to avoid as much as possible regular medication during pregnancy and delivery; and to let the child grow up as healthily as possible for at least the first two years.

One critical measure to insure a decrease in autism would be to postpone vaccination until age two and even then to reduce the number of vaccinations to a strict minimum. A second measure would be to make homeopathy and especially Isotherapy popular again all over the world to restore the energy of the mother and the father before pregnancy and help them avoid regular medication during pregnancy. If regular medicine is unavoidable, for example, when the mother has epilepsy or chronic colitis or other chronic diseases that need allopathic drugging, the child should be detoxified soon after his birth for these substances to clean his energy again and certainly before vaccinations are given.

The WHO and other child advocacy organizations should also stop the dangerous tetanus vaccinations during pregnancy as well as BCG and hepatitis B vaccinations at birth. A newborn child needs time and rest to adapt to this physical world without toxic injections from his first hours.

So what exactly is the process that leads to autism? In many cases it seems as if there is no process at all, but that is only appearance. The first causes that lead finally to the catastrophe of autism are invisible. When the child suddenly deteriorates it looks as if a certain vaccine or drug is responsible for the regression in his development. In seemingly all cases such events are just the last drop that makes the cup run over. The detoxification of this final event rarely gives complete healing. Studying the whole case from before the pregnancy up to that important event gives us all the other factors that have contributed to the final drama.

This also makes it understandable why some children can be born with autism. Their healing process has to be centered around events in the pregnancy or even before.

All this information, derived through the systematic application of Iso-therapy underscores the importance of being careful with the vulnerable brains of our future generations. Otherwise, the catastrophe will simply increase over the coming decades. Sadly, I see how these critical stages of life of our future generations have been assaulted by those who seek their own profit and do not understand or care for the healthy upbringing of our children. What we need are visionary and honest people, especially medical doctors, who have the courage to speak out against more and more vaccinations, additives in our food and toxins in our environment. Parents have to be informed with useful and correct information instead of being manipulated by the overblown fears promoted by corporations looking for their own profit.

How do we understand the accumulation of different causations? How is it possible that disturbances in the energetic field of a person accumulate? What is that exactly? First of all this idea is not an invention of my thinking, but simply an observation during the healing process of autistic children. As already stated earlier, even if the breakdown of the child clearly happens after a certain event, let us say, after the MMR, the detoxification of this MMR cannot completely heal the child again. This is an important observation. It suggests that there must already be other disturbances in the energy of the child that have allowed the MMR to give the final blow. But these other perturbations are of a different type and different energy. It could be for example a DTPP/Hib vaccine and an anti-emetic the mother took during the pregnancy.

How can these three causations accumulate? First of all, with all three of these causations the integrity of the energetic functioning of the child is disrupted. The energy of the child was not strong enough to keep a bad influence outside his system. Probably the immune system is involved here. Once there is a disruption in the energy, with a weakened immune system the next attack will more easily leave behind disturbing imprints. These disturbing energies go along with oxidative stress in the brain. Oxidative stress is in fact caused by free radicals of oxygen, which can disrupt all kinds of processes. That is why vitamin C is a powerful help in the reduction of this oxidative stress, especially ascorbyl palmitate (the fat-soluble form) because it easily bypasses the blood-brain barrier. So Vitamin C is protective against future damage, but it cannot heal toxic imprints in the child after they have already occurred.

This oxidative stress can cause a hyperactivation of the brain in general or of only certain parts of the brain. For that reason many autistic children are also gifted with qualities that normal children don't have; they are sometimes hyper intelligent or hyper performing. On the other side the energetic disturbances can also block the brain or parts of the brain and make its functioning difficult. Very often the part responsible for speech is blocked, and also the frontal lobe (responsible for the social/emotional life) is functioning in a survival mode. In addition, the motor area is often affected, causing the child to lag far behind in both his fine and gross motor skills.

Sometimes disturbing energies build up over time and release in the form of periodic epileptic attacks. It is easy to understand why 25% of autistic children have epileptic fits and 50% have an epileptic EEG. Following this same line of reasoning, we can also understand why in the same family one child is autistic and the other hyper intelligent. These hyper intelligent children live in a state before the breakdown. Apparently the brain has a threshold; when stress accumulates to the point that the balance is finally lost, epilepsy or a breakdown causing autism is the final outcome.

Let us see now a case which gives us some insight into the genesis of autism through the accumulation of different episodes of stress which leads finally to the fatal breakdown. As an aside, I never had this child under my treatment.

Case of a healthy baby becoming ill by medical intervention (vaccination and medication) in the first year

This case was sent to me by email and is a good example of what threatens the health and well-being of our future generations. [Comments in italics]

Hello Dr. Smits:

My story reads very much like many of the stories I have read throughout your PVS (post-vaccination syndrome) literature. I have an almost 3-year-old son, who was diagnosed with autism at 18 months of age after having received ALL of his vaccines. The following is the schedule of vaccines that Jim received:

2 days: Hep B
2 months: Infanrix Hexa + Prevnar (*7 different vaccines*)
3 ½ month: Prevnar, Hep B
5 months: Infanrix Hexa + Prevnar
7 months: Infanrix Hexa + Prevnar
9 months: Hep B
Between 7-9 months I noticed decreased speech and decreased receptiveness

At this stage there is already damage by the multiple vaccinations and his development and good health is already deteriorating.

9 months: yellowish mucus, eyelids shut, otitis media, pharyngitis. Rx: Amoxicillin (Antibiotic)

Here his vital energy tries to keep his integrity in balance as much as possible by the excretion of toxins through the eyes, ears and throat.

12 months: Otitis media
Rx: Amoxicillin

Discharge of toxins through the ears.

12 months: Varivax (varicella vaccine)
Started on milk; eczema and constant diarrhea

Now extra channels of excretion are used to drain the toxins after another vaccination.

14 months: Bilateral otitis media,
Rx: Amoxicillin
16 months: rashy, unresponsive, babbles, lost words (stopped saying MaMa and DaDa)

After the treatment of his otitis media with antibiotics the balance of his deteriorated health seems to be lost already and his brain cannot function normally any more, leading to impairment of important brain functions such as speech and social/emotional interactions.

16 months: MMR, Hib

The train of intoxication is not yet finished and no medical doctor seems to notice what is happening.

16 ¼ month: Otitis media,
Rx: Cefzil (Antibiotic)
16 ¾ month: Continued bilateral otitis media
Rx: Amoxicillin

Symptomatic treatment with antibiotics will not help him at all; what he needs is detoxification.

17 months: Not eating, rash on face

At this stage the body starts a new almost desperate attempt to survive and to detoxify — fasting.

17¾ month: Cranky; greenish drainage from nose, facial dermatitis, fungal sore on mouth, bilateral otitis.
Rx: Amoxicillin

His health is so bad now that fungus invades his mouth and the whole digestive system, aggravated by the use of regular courses of antibiotics; his skin is also affected; we see massive efforts to detoxify through the skin and both ears as well as deterioration of his mood.

18 months: diminished speech and receptiveness, eczema, DTaP

And if this was not yet enough he receives one more vaccine along with further deterioration of his general health and well-being.

18 months: Diagnosed with **autism**.

The painful reality of this diagnosis was, in some sense, inevitable. This reality can be seen daily all over the world. Why do we spoil our future generations with medical intervention? Why do we accept the systematic damaging of healthy children over the course of the first two years?

We have been to a million physicians along with one who follows the DAN protocol [Defeat Autism Now, a therapy involving many nutritional supplements]. We have Jim on a million supplements, a casein/gluten-free diet, DMSA, etc, ... but the treatment was unsuccessful.

Sure, many efforts are made by honest people, sometimes with good success, but the majority of these children will not be healed as long as we don't recognize that they are intoxicated, primarily by medical care itself; what they need, more than anything else is energetic detoxification to take off the energetic disturbances (imprints) that cause the malfunctioning of the whole system, mental, emotional and physical. Here homeopathy, in particular Isotherapy, is the medicine par excellence to do just that and bring the child back to a normal life again.

In this example I postulated that discharge from the ears, nose, throat and eyes can be interpreted as an attempt of the body's healing energy to detoxify the brain. In my view the mass of children that suffer repeated otitis media (ear infections) and chronic runny nose after vaccinations are a strong indication for this theory. In many little babies this detoxification starts shortly after the first or second shot. Strikingly, most children who are not vaccinated rarely have these infections.

Probably this explanation will not mesh with the ideas of doctors using regular medicine as their principal tool. They generally believe that an ear or throat infection is just a question of bacteria that develop because the immune system is not capable of stopping the development of these pathogenic bacteria. It is also believed that ear infections are normal because the Eustachian tube is still small in babies and that its function is not yet fully developed, creating a more or less closed cavity of the middle ear where the chance of infections is increased.

That these courses of antibiotics do not resolve the problem is clearly shown by the repeated necessity of their use. In other words, the more you give antibiotics the more these infections tend to recur. On the contrary, when the vaccines are detoxified with Isotherapy, these infections disappear like snow under the sun. This healing process seems to be accomplished first by restoring the child's functioning on the energetic level, and then on the physical level by strengthening the immune system and resolving oxidative stress. The immune system plays a vital role in protecting our brain against all kinds of damage. That is why we have to preserve our immune system like a precious jewel and even strive to make it more brilliant instead of damaging it with an excess of vaccines and other toxins. We have to change our medical thinking and practice, otherwise our future generations will have to face a deluge of children and adults damaged from autism, ADHD, aggressive behavior and chronic disabilities on the mental, emotional and physical level. We have to rethink what health is and how we can preserve it.

In the previous example we saw how the skin and the bowels (diarrhea) can be used as an extra outlet if the toxic pressure is too high. Through real healing therapy, which is in its essence not suppressive, this activation of outlets can be observed. When an appropriate homeopathic remedy has been administered in cases that need detoxification, the initial reaction is usually in the form of a discharge. The most common reactions are diarrhea, skin eruptions and runny nose, but also running ears or eyes are frequently seen. These reactions should by no means be suppressed with medications, but should be carefully guided by a professional homeopath, who knows how to interpret what happens and when it is necessary to support these excretions to avoid possible complications.

Antibiotics

Antibiotics are not as innocent as many people and doctors believe and can become a source of chronic disturbances. Certainly, antibiotics save many lives, but they also have another side. They don't just kill bacteria but weaken the immune system rather than reinforce it. Nevertheless, antibiotics are often considered as the sole solution to an infection. It is clear that a weakened immune system can only be reinforced by natural medicine, and homeopathy presents wonderful possibilities to do so.

The next case shows intoxication by antibiotics and how detoxification with a mixture of antibiotics in homeopathic doses heals that energetic imprint.

A case of intoxication with antibiotics

Very often the detoxification of antibiotics is part of the treatment of autistic children. Bart is a child whom I saw first in June 2007 and whose treatment was started with a detoxification course of antibiotics. He was five years old. At two years he was already behind in his development on the physical and mental/emotional level. He was quite aggressive, hitting, kicking, biting and pushing other children. With that he had a severe eczema that was treated unsuccessfully with all kinds of creams. He is diagnosed as autistic and retarded. At school he had become more and more unhappy, so the parents kept him home, looking for another school better suited for him. He was not able to dress and undress himself. He panicked easily when his life was not well structured and everything was not clear to him. He had to be prepared for everything. He did not accept contact with other children by himself. He was obsessed with moving and turning objects; he liked to turn the wheels of his toy cars. He retched when he got solid food in his mouth; his mother had to grind everything. His eczema was located on his wrists, around his mouth and on the back of his knees. He had had numerous colds with a sore throat, and his parents estimated that he had been given around *fifteen courses of antibiotics* starting from the age of one. His stool was solid. He had had strong night sweats for several years.

The pregnancy was uneventful, but the delivery was protracted. Ultimately, he was delivered by vacuum extraction. He got breast-feeding for only two months and had severe constipation, one stool every ten to fourteen days. At ten months his eczema started. At three and a half he had varicella (chicken pox). He wore glasses from age two on. He was very awkward and had rigid and obsessive behavior. His concentration was bad and he went from one place to another without being able to stay longer than a few seconds with a particular toy. He made contact easily. His speech developed slowly and he often repeated the same sentences. He had been vaccinated following the official program without special reactions.

I decided to start the treatment with the detoxification of his antibiotics. Therefore, he was given four dilutions of a mixture of different antibiotics: Poli-antibioticum 30C, 200C, 1M and 10M, every potency twice in a week, the whole course taking four weeks. Along with that he received Cuprum metallicum 30C once a week to resolve his rigidity and his obsessions along with vitamin C and fish oil.

During the first week he had a runny nose which is a good sign of detoxification of the brain. In homeopathy we say: 'The nose is the drain of the brain.' Even though Western medicine would not make this connection, our experience in homeopathy shows that the two often go together. In the second week his eczema became worse again (a typical sign that healing is occurring from the inside out, so it was no surprise that he then had cognitive and behavioral improvements). His concentration became better and he made longer sentences. He became potty-trained. He also stopped spinning in circles.

When the first signs of relapse appeared three weeks after the end of the detoxification of antibiotics, with bad concentration and unmanageable behavior, I decided to repeat the whole course for a second time. In the first week he had this same runny nose again and in the second week a worsening of his eczema. Then he remained stable much longer, for almost 2 months. His vision greatly improved in three months time and he no longer needed glasses. His concentration was better and he played nicely with his younger sister. His obsessions greatly diminished. When tired, especially in the evening, he was still aggressive, but his overall aggressiveness diminished a lot. A third detoxification course of Antibiotics was then given.

On the third course he progressed nicely: he was less obsessive, played with different toys and could sustain his concentration for 10 to 30 minutes instead of a few minutes. His speech was excellent. Nevertheless, there was still a lot to do. He was tired after school, although he had a good energy in the morning. He was very sensitive to too many people around him and his parents could not go to a party with him. He was still not able to dress and undress himself. The parents noticed that he had not been ill since the start of his detoxification therapy, whereas before he had had infections every three weeks. During the last course the eczema on his hands and on the back of his knees came back again. There are also still lags in his motor skills.

While he had already started to knock his head against the wall at 8 months and had a severe eczema at 12 months, the next step in the detoxification and healing process were his first vaccinations which were the DTPP and Hib, then the Neisvac-C and the MMR. The DTPP is given twice, the Neisvac-C 3 times and the MMR two times. Whether his eczema is better again the typical autistic features that are still there have not improved, so there must be still something else that we have overlooked and not treated yet. Presenting a checklist to the parents and with a list of his medication since his birth from the pharmacy we discovered that he was given frequently the nasal spray Xylomethazolin, which was already known to be causative in autism by means of the detoxifications in other children. He also got large quantities of hormonal crème with hydrocortisone.

After three months of breast feeding he was bottle fed with a plastic bottle heated up in the microwave until age three. So the treatment was first continued with the homeopathic preparation of xylomethazolin. On the 10M his eczema worsened again without finally giving the so wanted improvement. But he is more open, happier, has more fantasy and can concentrate longer. His motor skills are still far behind. Then he gets the homeopathic preparation of milk heated up in the microwave and after that the hydrocortisone has still to be detoxified. On the microwave milk treatment Bart had quite strong reactions especially on the 200C, but he improved again especially his eczema, which is almost completely gone for quite a time. His motor skills have improved a little bit, but at that point there is still much progress to make. He has also become calmer. The only detoxification that is programmed is the hydrocortisone, but the results are not yet known. When this book went to press, but his parents evaluated his overall healing at 75-80%. They emphasize also that during this two years of homeopathic treatment their son has never been ill any more, whereas before they had to go every two or three weeks to their family doctor.

Medication during pregnancy, increased risk for autism

Based on my understanding of the development of autism, it is of great importance to avoid medication during pregnancy and in the first two years. Unborn children and babies are not capable of handling toxins effectively. Therefore young children should not be vaccinated before 2 years of age. Furthermore it is advisable for parents to first observe the behavior and well-being of their baby and resolve any health problems, if need be, before beginning inoculations. I advise parents not to vaccinate their baby if he or she is ill or recovering from an illness; even a slight fever is a contraindication. In the chapter on vitamin C you will find the explanation for this.

A case of detoxifying medications taken during pregnancy

Pascal was three years old and his general development was severely retarded; he was already 21 months behind. His motor skills did not develop normally and his speech was restricted to a few single words. It was almost impossible to establish contact with him and he had no contact with other children. He salivated a lot and he needed his daily routine. His mother suffers from epilepsy and had used Depakin (valproic acid) during her pregnancy, which was tripled when she had an epileptic fit at five months. He was born with a vacuum extraction, although this should not disturb his development any more because it was treated at the time with osteopathy. He was vaccinated according to the official timetable. Around ten months he had varicella (chicken pox).

I started the treatment with the detoxification of the Valproic acid 30C, 200C, 1M and 10M, every potency four times in two weeks in a course of eight weeks. Along with that he was given the usual fat soluble vitamin C (ascorbyl palmitate) three times a day 1 gram, an ascorbate (water soluble vitamine C) with zinc and magnesium 500mg three times a day, and 500mg of fish oil per day. Shortly after this first detoxification the eye contact was clearly better; he was more open and his stature was more upright. He stopped putting his fingers or other things constantly in his mouth. He also showed more affection, spontaneously sitting close to his mother.

Subsequently, I repeated the eight week course. After this second course he continuously progressed. His social skills improved considerably and he liked to cuddle now with his parents. If I ask the parents what is the overall result of these past five months of therapy they say there is remarkable progress on all levels and that he has far more personality now.

Another typical example: detoxification with a classical homeopathic treatment

Robbert is the prototype of a child that we see so often these days. Up to age one and a half he was an almost trouble-free, healthy child developing normally. Then not only did his normal progress stop, but in many ways he began to regress. His smoothly developing speech disappeared, and he became clumsy and started to have a lot of behavior problems. He flapped his hands when excited and walked on tiptoes. He could suddenly erupt with rage was hypersensitive to noises and, finally, his ability to make eye contact disappeared. Ultimately, his alertness and happiness vanished.

I saw him at three and a half after he had been diagnosed as autistic. In his past history there were some unmistakable indications that his balance was already disturbed before he was one and a half. In his first year he had several bouts of otitis media, as well as severe constipation, requiring occasional use of a laxative. After age one he suffered asthmatic respiration, necessitating prophylactic Ventolin and Pulmicort. Any time he had a runny nose there were complications. At one and a half he had surgery to put tubes in his ears along with removal of his adenoids. All this indicated that the early vaccinations could have been causative in this case. Therefore I started his treatment with the systematic detoxification of the vaccines he had received so far. First he was given Neisvac-C (Meningococ-C) in 4 potencies every potency twice in a two week course. Then after one week's rest the MMR was given over four weeks and finally the DTTP/Hib over 4 weeks as well. Three months later the first round of detoxification was finished.

The DTPP/Hib course provoked the strongest reactions. During the course his behavior became worse and he was extremely irritable. But the results were very satisfying. The most striking improvements were in his speech and understanding. He could make sentences up to five words and his comprehension greatly increased. Also his gaze was much more open and his behavior with other children became more social. He became the most teachable child of his group. At his kindergarten they called him a prodigy.

Then a second course of DTPP/Hib was given, again over four weeks. After that he really started to express himself verbally and his vocabulary increased markedly. He used his toys appropriately and his imagination grew enormously. His obsessions gradually decreased.

His immune system became much stronger. The Ventolin and Pulmicort were stopped and when he had a runny nose there were no complications any more. His constipation was also better, but not completely gone.

A third course of DTPP/Hib did not give further improvements, so the treatment was continued with the next step, which in his case is the activation of his neocortex with a homeopathic remedy. I prescribed Saccharum off. 30C, twice a week, to stimulate his social/emotional skills and Saccharum off. D6 daily to ameliorate his digestion. Such a switch to a constitutional remedy can be very effective, under the express condition that all detoxifications have been executed first. If the treatment with a constitutional remedy tends to be successful at the beginning but proves to become ineffective in higher potencies there is a strong indication that some imprint has not been corrected yet. That is exactly what happened in this case.

Over the five months that he took this medication he progressed markedly. His speech became more and more natural. He could make sentences of three to five words. He started to eat what was cooked and tried more varied foods, including vegetables and fruit. It was as if a button has been pushed, his mother said. For the first time I could have a little conversation with him during the consultation, despite the prediction of his previous doctors that he would never talk. He was still quite obsessive with numbers and letters and sometimes had tantrums. The healing was evaluated by the parents at 60%. The healing process continued during the next half year with Saccharum 200C, but his lack of flexibility, his tendency to control everything and his intolerance to changes, which made him a little dictator, became more prominent. This I have often seen during treatment with Saccharum. It is the Cuprum part of autism that becomes stronger. Saccharum cannot heal this. Nowadays I give Saccharum and Cuprum in alternation, and it works wonderfully in avoiding these kinds of aggravations. At this point in the treatment, I combined the Saccharum 1M with Cuprum metallicum 30C, but his reaction on the Cuprum was not good. His hypersensitivity, especially in his mouth, came back; he started to lick everything; his anger increased again with shouting and physical aggression, including biting and pinching. He complained of being tired and fearful. This reaction on Cuprum is unusual. It meant that some disturbance was still there that could not be lifted by Cuprum. After reflection and investigation my interpretation was that the vaccines were still not fully detoxified, so I decided to once again give courses of Neisvac-C, MMR and DTPP/Hib. The Neis-vac-C provoked no reaction at all with no improvement; during the MMR course he had a lot of reactions: he was angry, very rigid, tear-ful and weak. The DTTP/Hib course caused only a slight reaction.

Subsequently, he was more manageable and less hypersensitive. He did his best to control his aggression, and he was more open to his mother. He started telling her what bothered him and that was new. But I felt this was not really the solution. Certainly, he had made some progress through the detoxification, but there was no real break-through.

Over that last half year I became more and more aware that often medication during and even before pregnancy was the basis for autism. Regardless of whether I had written in a child's file that the pregnancy and delivery were uneventful, I would reinvestigate it. At this point the mother told me that she had frequent and often quite severe attacks of colic during her pregnancy and used Buscopan (butylcopolamine) and Diclofenac. This latter should normally not be used during pregnancy, and she even had high doses of it. In the last month of her pregnancy her mother died and to help with her grief (which is also stress for the child) she took Oxazepam. With this information it will probably be possible to heal the last 30%, which, according to the parents, is what was still left. So the treatment is continued with Oxazepam 30C, 200C, 1M and 10M, every potency twice over 4 weeks. Then the Diclofenac is detoxified, same poten-cies and treatment and finally Buscopan with a two-week interval between each treatment. But these three treatments did not give any improvement. Furthermore, their younger son has also autism and has not been vaccinated. The only conclusion is and can be that some other factor has provoked autism in both her children. It is important to find these causative factors to make the healing process complete. The parents had already accepted that these positive results of 70% healing is the maximum we could achieve with Robbert, but it is not. If also their second son is autistic it is probable that there is a common factor that was already present before the pregnancy. I have sent them a checklist now. The use of a checklist of possible causative factors has greatly improved our ability to gather all the information at the first consultation.

A case of detoxifying medication during the first two years of life
I want to show this case because it demonstrates nicely that autism is an accumulation of different causes and that Isotherapy is able to detect these causes and eliminate them.

Up to 30 months of age, Rob was a happy and contented child with kidney problems, which were diagnosed during pregnancy. At birth his kidneys were already under stress because the urine flowed back from his bladder to his kidneys (reflux). Therefore he was immediately given prophylactic antibiotics and a renogram was performed. In his first year of life these renograms were repeated six times, and once he was catheterized while on antibiotics. He was vaccinated like all other children in the Netherlands with DTPP/Hib, Neisvac-C, MMR and even got an extra hepatitis A shot at age four. Up to two and a half years he showed no noticeable problems, but from that time forward he started to speak more and more slowly. When the whole family moved to another house, the parents believed he had some difficulties adapting to the new situation. Finally, at age four even the children's health center admitted that something was wrong.

At school he was unable to concentrate, was absent-minded, had difficulty interacting with other children, could not tolerate too many stimuli and was unable to stand up for himself in the group. His development had slowed down.

When I first saw 6-year-old Rob he already had severe problems. His voice was loud, staccato, monotone and stilted. He had an obsessive interest in animals and was restless, talking continuously and jumping and running excessively. He had no boundaries. He approached people too closely and held objects too closely to their face when he wanted to show something. His fine and gross motor skills were weak.

At home he was quite obedient and slept well. He could stay angry for a long time and needed strict rules and structure. He could show some empathy, but not at school. His provisional diagnosis was Asperger's.

I started his treatment with Saccharum off. 30C and Cuprum metallicum 30C, both once a week, ascorbyl palmitate and an ascorbate complex 1000mg with magnesium and zinc three times per day and fish oil three times daily. I noted in the margin of my file that he had to be detoxified for MMR, Neisvac-C, DTPP/Hib and the fluid used for the renogram. After three months there were some changes. He recovered much quicker from his anger and was more able to play with other children. On the other hand he had become very restless and showed no boundaries at all in what he was saying to other people. He flapped his hands when he was excited. His sensitivity to taste and smell had dramatically increased. He could not tolerate butter near him; even the sight of it made him retch. He developed a strong aversion for eggs, cheese and butter, but adored milk, fish and meat.

I decided to start right away with the detoxification, because continuing the actual treatment would probably not give the desired results. First Neisvac-C was given in homeopathic potencies. During the first course he was very restless; during the second he developed a strong diarrhea, which indicated a good detoxification. At the third course there was no further reaction. He immediately made a great leap forward at school. His concentration span improved from 3 minutes to 40 minutes and at the end of the school year he was allowed to stay at a regular school with some extra counseling.

At the MMR he had no reactions, so the DTPP/Hib was started. On the 30C his face swelled up, his eyes, lips and even his tongue. His mother phoned me and I advised her to give him 2 granules of the DTTP/Hib 30C in a glass of water, a sip every hour which generated a quick improvement. She then repeated the 30C during the summer holidays and was amazed to see him tinker with scissors, glue and clay, which he had never done before. The DTTP/Hib course was repeated three times with frequent repetitions of each potency because of the many reactions. After this his mother told me that she was amazed that the treatment had such an impact on him. Not everybody in their circle of acquaintance was convinced when the parents told them what had happened to their son; it just seemed too far-fetched. The father was really amazed that it worked at all. He had lost a little brother from the smallpox vaccination.

Rob made progress by leaps and bounds. His motivation improved markedly and at school he was doing well. He no longer stayed by himself on the playground; nevertheless, he continued to seem as if he was playing next to children and not with them. He sang, laughed and frolicked happily. He was now able to listen and his speech was less affected. His anger disappeared in large part and he was able to say he was sorry. The parents estimated his overall improvement at 50-60%. His main problems were: his sensitivity to stimuli, his incapacity to separate main issues from side-issues and his intolerance for large groups like at parties.

The next step I took was the detoxification of the many renograms he had had in his first year of life. The fluid that was used for them contained tin chloride and technetium. Because it took some time to get the Technetium in homeopathic potencies, I once again put Rob on Saccharum 200C and Cuprum metallicum 200C. Despite this, after two months he had a general relapse after he travelled with his parents to Egypt.

Then the Stannum muriaticum (tin chloride) course was started and that was the point that I wanted to get with this case. Chemical substances, especially during the first years can have a strong impact on the brain functions.

He had strong reactions to every potency of Stannum muriaticum, which suggests that the energetic disturbances had infected the four different levels of his energy. He was angry, unreachable and unfocused: he made many noises and was no longer able to stop his emotional outbursts. This type of worsening sometimes happens during the vaccine clearing. It is difficult for the parents to witness so I have to keep reminding them that it is part of the healing process. If the child does not react at all, there can be no progress. If there is a strong reaction, even a negative one, it means the child is having a profound response to the vaccine clearing, which can lead to great progress after the course has ended. So sometimes parents need encouragement to stay the course and complete the vaccine clearing when the child has a reaction like this. Rob received every potency twice the number of times of the usual repetitions, i.e. each potency was administered four times. After this course he started to improve again. He was able to really play and interact with other children. He was open to arguments again and exhibited more self-reflection and self-consciousness. He was also able to stop playing when it was time to eat.

Surprisingly, there was no reaction on the Technetium course. That simply meant that the technetium was not in any way responsible for his autism. So the Stannum muriaticum course was repeated a second time, which made him angry and restless once again. After that course he improved again. He realized that he was different from other children. He now maintained the appropriate physical distance from other children. He was able to understand jokes and his motor skills improved. He was less obsessive and had more different interests. He showed more empathy. But when the place was too crowded he lost his concentration and he was still not able to understand the interaction in children's games.

Now a third course of Stannum muriaticum has to be given to get the maximum out of this detoxification, and his hepatitis A and antibiotics detoxification are still on the program. Much has been done so far and there is a good chance of complete healing for Rob when we finally have gone through all the necessary steps to get his energy flowing again unhindered.

Hypersensitivity

Most autistic children suffer from some kind of hypersensitivity to sounds, light, textures, taste and smells. This, from my perspective, is due to the oxidative stress which makes certain parts of the brain hyperactive. The next story illustrates this concept. I asked Gabriel's parents to tell the story themselves. When I had the mother on the phone ten weeks after the start of my therapy, she was very enthusiastic about Gabriel's progress. I prescribed Saccharum 30C and Cuprum metallicum 30C with the two kinds of vitamin C and fish oil. When I asked how much better Gabriel was, she said 99%. As you will discover there is still a lot to be healed, but life became so much happier for all of them, that it felt like almost 100%. Here is his story.

Testimonial of Gabriel's parents

In July of 2006, we lived in genuine despair; we had no idea how we could help Gabriel. He had started to have very frequent panic attacks as never before, almost one every 30 minutes. His senses seemed to be amplified a thousand times. We, his parents, could not make the slightest sound or even speak around him; sometimes even our breathing made him go into an uncontrollable panic attack, where he would be very hard to manage or comfort. Within the family, we avoided saying certain words or sounds; we avoided even speaking to each other in front of Gabriel. We came to the point of spending several days in silence, at home and outside. He would only tolerate gestures; even coughing would send him into a state of panic.

Certain sounds from the television, even songs or toys which before he had seemed to prefer, became terrifying to him. Even the light from the sunset that came through our living room windows was intolerable for him.

Gabriel's mother always had to be visible to him. Even in the home, she could not be in another room. This made simple things like going to the bathroom or doing simple household chores extremely difficult.

When we would go out, we were the ones to follow Gabriel, rather than he following our lead. We would always choose carefully the locations (fields, parks, beaches, etc.), so he would be able to walk and explore as freely as possible. Gabriel was always very difficult to guide, even holding his hand. It was always extremely difficult to stop and rest, as the act of waiting was impossible. At his grandparent's house, he would only tolerate being there less than a half hour. In August and September, his panic attacks grew in frequency and intensity. We began to suspect that these attacks were due to strong headaches, which caused screaming and sweating around his head, and only stopped when he was so tired that he would fall asleep. We consulted a neurologist, who did an MRI. The result was that everything was normal, no problem. As a precaution, the neurologist prescribed Tegretol, an anti-epileptic drug, which was also supposed to calm him. It helped him for a week or so, but then his crisis continued. In October we travelled to the U.S., for Gabriel's third appointment at the Pfeiffer Treatment Center. Returning from the

U.S., Gabriel seemed better. The Pfeiffer Treatment Center suggested some nutrients to calm Gabriel, such as GABA, Inositol and 5-HTP.

They helped very much, and Gabriel's crisis diminished drastically. Only his agitation persisted, with much sweating from very little activity. In November he started going to pre-school in the mornings, a great new challenge for him, because of his behavior, learning difficulties and health problems.

In December of 2006, when Gabriel was five we consulted Dr. Tinus Smits and initiated his homeopathic and nutritional treatment. After 6 months, Gabriel is a more confident child, not only with us, his mother and father, but also with other adults, such as other family members, therapists and teachers. He still has many difficulties in sitting, paying attention and learning simple tasks, for some minutes. His constant tantrums or panic attacks, which occurred night and day, disappeared. As he grew more confident and aware, he became more flexible and tolerant of his surroundings. Now, he's normally always in a good mood, exploring more of the world around him and vocalizing more and more sounds and songs. When he suffers from his chronic intestinal problems or headaches, he now accepts our comforting and consoling him. He adores when we play with him and make him laugh, and he is more and more affectionate. He loves to share his play activities with us, especially playing catch. He loves to go out to the park, and now he seeks to play with other children or see what they're doing. Of course, other children don't understand him, mainly because of his disorder: his language delays and his stereotypical body movements (hypersensitivities). But he is a child with an admirable vital energy.

We're convinced that Gabriel will recuperate even further, especially from the damages of vaccination, with the continuation of this most appropriate treatment.

Different causations

From my understanding three routes of causation for autism can be considered:

1. **Stress factors after birth** due to vaccinations; repeated courses of antibiotics due to recurring infections; anesthesia and other medications; and toxicity from plastic softeners, aspartame, glutamate, etc.

2. **Toxic factors during pregnancy:** emotional stress and/or physical stress due to medication of the mother with anti-epileptics, anti-pyretics, or other drugs, smoking, alcohol and/or junk-food with low vitamin C intake. In many of these cases vaccinations or toxic factors after birth are just the final stimulus. Every medication during pregnancy has to be considered as potentially harmful for the unborn child. A difficult or premature birth can also have a harmful effect. These children should be seen by an osteopath or cranio-sacral therapist as well. A blocked cranium can cause tremendous tension.

3. **Toxic factors in the parents before conception:** vaccinations against tropical diseases, hepatitis B and/or a repetition of their DTP; parents who had Lyme disease, mononucleosis, fibromyalgia, inhalers for asthma, medication for arthritis or for other infectious diseases; parents that are under chronic medication; parents who have bad food habits with the intake of bad oils, low omega-3 fatty acids, lots of sugar and low vita-min C intake and who are smokers or alcohol drinkers.

CHAPTER 5

DETOXIFICATION OF VACCINES USING
POTENTIZED VACCINES

One of the wonderful applications of the homeopathic principle is the use of the same diluted and potentized substances that have caused damage in the human body. In classical homeopathy we face the difficulty of finding the right remedy based on the symptoms and our understanding of the patient. When we use potentized substances which caused damage, commonly called Isotherapy, the match with the causative factor is perfect. This is what makes Isotherapy so effective. The primary problem is to find the different causative factors without omitting any of them. This method is one of the pillars of my treatment of autism.

A case of great progress with vaccine detoxification
Some years ago I received this e-mail from the US. It shows nicely what this technique of detoxification can accomplish in the treatment of autistic children.

Hello Dr. Smits,

I read your website with great interest. My son (now 29 months) became severely autistic with other biological health issues after his first DTPol shot. We have seen a classical homeopath with great success over the past 13 months. This past dose of DTPol remedy has been nothing short of a miracle. In quick summary, my son went from a child that did not speak, did not play, did not interact, banged his head repeatedly all day, spun in circles and other stims, suffered leaky gut syndrome, yeast infections, and other issues, to a little boy who now speaks, plays, laughs, is potty trained, and by all other measures is a normal toddler. There are no residual autistic symptoms! However, he must remain on a strict diet. He can only eat rice, potato, pears, chicken and beef. He can also tolerate sheep's yogurt. He is still very intolerant of gluten, casein, soy, corn and phenols.

Isotherapy can also be used to exclude possible causative factors. When there is doubt if a certain vaccine has caused damage, giving the vaccine in 30C, 200C, 1M and 10M can bring clarity. If there is hardly any reaction and there is no change in the health status after the detoxification course, you can be sure there must be something else that is responsible for the persisting symptoms. Isotherapy can be used as a diagnostic tool in this way. For example, Lyme is difficult to detect. If blood tests for Lyme are negative, but there is suspicion that Lyme is present, then successful treatment with the Lyme detoxification protocol will confirm the presence of the disease.

To understand how detoxification works, we have to consider that diseases are not only caused by substances like bacteria, viruses, fungi, toxic matters, etc., as is the main belief in conventional medicine, but that *every substance can also cause an imprint in the energetic field of a person.* These imprints are not only from direct damage to the person, e.g. by vaccination, a disease (influenza, mononucleosis, etc.), emotional trauma (death of a child, divorce, etc.), but can also be transmitted from the parents to the unborn child.

Vaccinations can cause very profound disturbances and can be transmitted from one generation to another. It is not the disease itself or the causative substance that is transmitted, but rather the energetic imprint in the energetic field of the future father and the mother.

Case of the parents' vaccines as partial causation

Recently I saw an eight-year-old autistic boy who has been under my treatment for two years and has greatly benefited from the detoxification of vaccines, as well as homeopathic and orthomolecular treatment. In fact, he has become in two years time a normal boy, except for his speech. During these two years there was no improvement in his clumsy speech. He was only able to talk in two to three word phrases and unable to pronounce more difficult words. I reconsidered the whole case to find out what could cause the blockage in his speech center. I worked to discover why his speech didn't improve while all the rest was better. There was no event in his eight years of life that we had overlooked; even the pregnancy was uneventful. Nevertheless, there was one striking fact that put me on the track. Both parents were working for years at the KLM airline as pursers and got many vaccinations before the child was born. Could the damage that the vaccinations of the parents caused in their energy have been transmitted to their future child? As I stated, the father and mother can transmit not only their genetic shortcomings, but also their energetic disturbances. So I studied their vaccination status before conception and prescribed two courses of detoxification to the boy, the first one typhoid and the second one yellow fever. On both he had quite strong reactions, and to the parents' and my delight, after these detoxifications his speech improved greatly and for the first time in his life, he was able to speak like almost any other boy of his age. I was surprised myself.

A case of reversing the mother's illness prior to pregnancy

Another story, which has nothing to do with autism, can also serve to clarify this energetic transmission of the parents' health problems. I saw in my consulting room a five-month-old baby who was on antibiotics from birth. She had already had pneumonia or almost pneumonia three times. Her lungs were full of mucus, and she had a chronic cough and rattling respiration. The mother was desperate. Fortunately, she postponed the vaccines, wanting her daughter to be healthy before starting with them. My own process of reasoning led me to conclude that if this little girl was born with a poorly functioning immune system, the causation should be sought before birth. But the delivery and the pregnancy were uneventful. The mother even felt better during pregnancy and she never took any medications. So I asked her how she was at the start of her pregnancy. She said: 'Oh, I was tired. I had been tired for 10 years already. At age twenty I got mononucleosis quite severely. I was home for a whole year and never recovered fully.' I prescribed a course of Mononucleosis (prepared as a homeopathic remedy) over 15 days for the baby. She recovered dramatically. After two weeks the mucus and rattling respiration and her chronic colds were gone and her immune system was able to function normally.

Because of these experiences I now look much more carefully at what happened in the lives of the parents before the conception of the child. What we can also learn from these cases is that very specific causations can be involved in the process of becoming autistic, and that homeopathy has the perfect tools in its potentized equivalents of these causations to treat them successfully. It also teaches us that there is hardly ever one causation, but that there is an accumulation of stress-provoking factors that together contribute to the genesis of autism.

Different energetic levels

Another aspect of this energetic transfer is that the imprints can be located at different energetic levels, depending on how deeply the disturbance entered the energetic field of the patient. Thus, some patients react strongly on the 30C and hardly at all on the higher potencies, while others react mainly on the higher potencies. Usually, the reaction is the strongest on just one or two potencies of the series that is given, but it is not exceptional to see reactions at every potency. To completely heal these imprints it is important to use the 30C, 200C, 1M and the 10M, each of which corresponds to a different energetic level. These four potencies cover in general the entire field where the disturbance has taken place. Nevertheless, in exceptional cases lower (6 and 12) or higher potencies (50M, i.e., 50,000C) may be required.

How to administer these different potencies

The duration of a course to detoxify a serious health problem is typically one month, every week a different potency with every potency administered twice, e.g., on Monday and Thursday. Deep-seated disturbances should not be treated with short courses. In serious cases like epilepsy, it is wise to use an eight-week scheme, repeating every potency four times. It is important to observe the reactions from each potency and never to go to a higher potency when there are still reactions from the previous potency to avoid overly strong detox reactions and to erase the disturbance completely at that energetic level. All kinds of detoxification reactions may occur. The most common are eliminative reactions with an increase of reactivity (fever). Fever should not be treated with medication, as it is a healthy reaction of the organism and not a disease! It helps greatly to overcome an acute disturbance, shortens the healing process, stimulates reactivity and avoids complications. Eliminations like diarrhea, flu, expectoration, and bad-smelling and cloudy urine should also be left alone, because they are a part of the healing process.

A case of diarrhea as a cleansing reaction

I remember an autistic child who got diarrhea during the detoxification of his vaccines. The diarrhea relieved his system so much, that his autism almost disappeared instantly. After ten days the mother started to worry and went to the family doctor because I was absent at that moment. He prescribed Imodium (Loperamide) to stop the diarrhea by paralyzing the peristaltic motions of the bowels. Almost immediately the child had a setback and became autistic as before. The diarrhea was a perfect detoxification for his bowels and brain.

Neither the doctor nor the mother understood this, and the medication interfered with the progress of the cure.

Between different courses of detoxification, a two week rest should be inserted to let the detoxification finish its work and to see if the new situation is stable. If there is a relapse during this pause the same detoxification should be started earlier.

A long run of detoxification may also be followed by a short one to test whether the detoxification has been effectuated completely. The mistake parents often make is the application of the basic schedule without the extra repetitions when the child starts to react. When this happens the course has to be repeated as before with emphasis on the continued administration of the same potency whenever there is a reaction.

The administration is carried out by letting two granules melt in the mouth. Such a treatment should never be executed by the parents themselves; it should be managed by an experienced homeopath who is familiar with the detoxification of vaccines and other substances. The success of such a treatment depends greatly on the correct interpretation of what happens during the detoxification. The 'CEASE Autism' organization is working hard to create certified homeopaths worldwide to insure that a high quality of treatment is guaranteed and parents will not be disappointed. You can find these certified practitioners on our website www.cease-autism.com.

Unnoticed vaccination damage

The diagnosis of vaccination damage is not always obvious. Many conventional and even some complementary doctors are not used to perceiving the relationship between certain complaints and earlier shots. There are quite a number of cases where subtle observation and investigation are necessary to come to the right conclusion. Eline developed a cough subsequent to her first vaccination which pointed in that direction, but even the parents were not aware that these same shots had damaged her overall wellbeing.

Eline is an apparently healthy child of five years, but she had already started to cough in her first year. Her lungs were always full of mucus, and she had a paroxysmal suffocative cough at night. In the summertime she had hardly any problem. Her energy was quite low for a five-year-old and she sucked her thumb frequently during the day. After eating she was tired. She regularly had fever, especially when the cough was severe. Six months ago she even had convulsions with the fever. She was a difficult and slow eater, disliked warm food and hardly ate any vegetables. She drank little and was fond of sweets. Almost every night she slipped into her parents' bed and had a difficult start in the morning. She had good social contacts and was an easygoing and reasonable child without tantrums.

Her mother almost drowned when she was four months pregnant. Eline was only breastfed a few days due to cracks in her mother's nipples, but the bottle-feeding was without problems. At two months she got her first vaccination, and a few days later the cough started.

If we look to the cause of her problem, her first vaccination was almost certainly the origin of her cough. So I prescribed DTPP/Hib 30C, 200C, 1M and 10M, every potency twice over a period of four weeks. Her cough then disappeared almost completely. After a two week interval a second course was given to finish the cough 100%. Indeed, her cough then disappeared completely, but more striking was her emotional growth. She became quite sure of herself, more active, more responsible and her school results improved considerably. Although her energy was much better, it was not yet optimal. Therefore a third course was given. Then the disturbing energy from the DTPP/Hib shot was definitely erased from her energetic system and was no longer capable to disturb her vital functions. She recovered completely and had a good energy again.

A case illustrating the repetition of single potencies.

The following case shows the overwhelming results of the detoxification of only one vaccine over a period of ten months. Here the principle of repeating a potency as long as there are reactions has been correctly applied, thereby altering the standard course of four weeks to a course of ten months. Even after this long course, an additional short course had to be given to test whether there was still any disturbance left from that shot. The lack of reaction to this final course verified that all disturbance had been thoroughly eradicated from his energetic system.

Jimmy was almost four years old when I first saw him in a consultation with his mother and grandparents. The father left the mother when Jimmy was 6 months old. Jimmy had been diagnosed autistic at a young age and his mother had already tried treating him in an early stage because his speech was not developing. Two and a half years of frustration followed, because no institute was able to help her son.

His mother had a difficult pregnancy. She felt tired, lonely and abandoned. She endured a lot of fights with her husband. She remembered that she had wept almost constantly over the last months. Her son was born at 35 and a half weeks. The delivery was induced because she had started to swell up almost as if the tears could not come out any more. The first year of his life was like so many other babies. He was breastfed for four months. Although he had frequent regurgitations up to age eight or nine months, his overall development was appropriate. After his first DTPP/Hib/Hep-B (HEXA) at three months he had a severe diarrhea, refused to eat and was flabby. After the MMR at 15 months he developed a chronic diarrhea that subsided only a few months before I saw him. In the first year he had several middle ear infections, always right-sided, with frequent courses of antibiotics.

With the overload of the current vaccination program, these kinds of histories are not exceptional anymore. His energy was desperately trying to restore the balance. Both his ears and his bowels became efficient outlets for the system to get rid of the poison. But shortly after the MMR the balance was finally and permanently disturbed, and the brain was put in survival mode, stopping normal development on the mental, emotional and physical levels.

He had the typical symptoms that are common in autistic children. He said two or three words without purpose, but was able to understand almost everything. There was no eye contact any more. If he did not get what he wanted, he struck his mother and tore at her hair. He was very impatient and hyperactive. He was hypersensitive to noise and could hardly play with other children. His intelligence seemed not to have suffered too much; his understanding was not too bad and he had an excellent memory and could follow instructions. He had progressed a lot already when his mother started to give him fish oil one year before I saw him. Within two weeks there was a clear overall amelioration.

The treatment started with homeopathic HEXA (the shot is a combination of diphtheria, tetanus, whooping cough, polio, Hib and hepatitis B). I gave the usual instructions with this treatment, which included giving every potency twice weekly and not moving to a higher potency if the second dose still elicited reactions. If there are no clear reactions the whole course is finished in four weeks. With those instructions they disappeared from my view for almost a year.

Jimmy had quite strong reactions at every administration whatever the potency. So all the potencies were repeated 6 to 10 times, the whole course lasting ten months. He started right away with high fever and diarrhea with bloody and very dark-colored and cloudy urine; he felt miserable. He got several spots of eczema, which he also had before. This all meant an enormous reactivation of his vital energy and a fantastic process of detoxification and healing. Old symptoms came back: he started biting himself again, walked on his tip-toes, squinted again and got red ears, especially on the right side where he had had his repeated ear infections. And with all this he became very angry and difficult to handle. His mother started to doubt herself, wondering if she had taken the wrong path for treating her son. Nevertheless, her doubts evaporated, because she began noticing that the stronger the detox reactions the more her son progressed.

After ten months the results were considerable. The greatest joy for his mother was the first time he intentionally said, 'Mama'; she burst into tears. At the follow-up, Jimmy could correctly use *I* and *you* and was able to explain his own thoughts. The eye contact was back again and he could make contact with other children and play with them. He could once again engage in fantasy play. He intentionally looked around and observed the world around him. He was awake and alert and his fits of anger had diminished tenfold. He was able to express different states of mood like sadness and joy. He learned by himself to count up to thirty and recognized them if they were written. He was interested in learning the alphabet. At school his teacher was astonished by his progress. His restlessness was much better, but he was still quite an active child. When I asked the mother how she evaluated the whole process, she said: 'This is 20 times better than I had hoped.'

CHAPTER 6

VITAMIN C

My interest in vitamin C stems from the cancer therapy which I developed, *Non-Toxic Tumor Therapy*. Here vitamin C plays an important role as an antioxidant. In addition to always using water-soluble vitamin C, fat-soluble vitamin C (ascorbyl palmitate) is often prescribed, particularly in brain tumors. Vitamin C also seems to play an essential role in protecting children against the adverse effects of vaccinations or other stress-inducing events. This was demonstrated by the Australian doctor Dr. Archie Kalokerinos, who witnessed a twofold increase in child mortality among Aboriginals after vaccination campaigns. Because human beings are unable to produce vitamin C themselves and therefore totally depend on vitamin C intake, extra vitamin C is necessary in stress situations such as vaccinations, infections or other diseases, and emotional stress. When Dr. Kalokerinos started giving vitamin C to Aboriginal children, he was able to reduce child mortality, at the time about 50%, to practically zero. (As a side note, Dr. Kalokerinos also advises against the vaccination of sick or not yet fully recovered children. In the Netherlands, authorities have grossly overlooked this and almost never postpone vaccinations when a child is not completely healthy. I even saw a baby with severe brain damage, still struggling for his life after the first shot, who got his second vaccination in an academic hospital, just because it was time for his second vaccination.)

Dr. Kalokerinos' work has led me to prescribe vitamin C as a preventive measure. Then when I witnessed that autism often improved by detoxifying the vaccines, I thought vitamin C could not only be useful in *preventing* autism from vaccinations, but that it could possibly play an important part in *curing* it as well. When I first prescribed ascorbyl palmitate (the fat-soluble vitamin C) for a four-year-old autistic child, both his speech and comprehension improved dramatically. His mother was deeply impressed by the significant improvement. Since then, ascorbyl palmitate has played an essential part in my treatment protocol for autistic children.

Vitamin C is known to have many effects on the human body, which could be very relevant for autistic children:

1. Vitamin C neutralizes harmful oxidants (oxidative stress) such as the hydroxyl radical (OH^-) and regenerates Vitamin E for reuse.

2. When vitamin C takes part in anti-oxidative processes, the ascorbate radicals that are produced are relatively harmless and are easily recycled into active ascorbates

3. Vitamin C stimulates the excretion of copper and thus aids in the reduction of stress. All autistic children have elevated copper levels as has been documented by the Pfeiffer Treatment Center, Naperville, Illinois.

4. Vitamin C also stimulates the elimination of heavy metals, such as mercury, lead, cadmium and nickel.

5. Vitamin C is required for the formation of L-carnitine, which in turn is necessary within the cell for the normal use of fats for energy

6. Vitamin C aids folate metabolism by the transformation of folic acid into folinic acid.

7. Vitamin C loosens the stool in severely constipated children and stimulates the intestine; too high a dose may cause diarrhea, but is otherwise harmless.

These are just some of the known effects, and there must be many more still unknown effects of this miraculous vitamin.

Vitamin C and other supplements

For everybody who has studied the orthomolecular approach to autism, which supplements to give is an important and difficult question. Many parents have their child checked for deficiencies and toxins. Typically, the more detailed the research, the more is discovered. Also allergies (e.g., gluten and casein) are very common in autistic children. Supplementation, however, has its limits. It is true that some supplements have given miraculous results in a few autistic children, but when applied to other children the results were disappointing. I also tried supplements such as lipoic acid, glutathione, cystein, glutamic acid, l-carnitine, MSM, etc. To be sure, I did not test them extensively, but all these supplements worked only if combined with the rest of my treatment. Gradually, I omitted all these supplements and nowadays I use only the water- and fat-soluble vitamin C combined with extra zinc and magnesium. Vitamin C, by virtue of its strong power of reduction, helps a number of other processes to work better. Even without considering the financial burden, it is my opinion that to administer a lot of supplements to heal the child is not always the best solution.

Water- and/or fat-soluble vitamin C

Vitamin C does not enter the brain easily since the brain barrier is permeable only to fat-soluble substances. In this way the brain is protected against toxic materials. By using the fat-soluble form of vitamin C (ascorbyl palmitate), it is possible to transport a larger amount of vitamin C to the brain. To prevent the body from using too large an amount of this fat-soluble vitamin C elsewhere, or from transforming it into water-soluble vitamin C, I always make sure to prescribe the water-soluble vitamin C. I use it in the ascorbate form. This is the non-acidic form bound to a mineral like calcium, potassium, magnesium or zinc. This enables the administration of minerals in combination with the vitamin C. The non-acidic vitamin C is generally better tolerated. A very important, perhaps even the most important function of vitamin C in the brain is the reduction of oxidative stress. This is accomplished by clearing away free radicals and by methylating various substances. In the US, methyl-cobalamine (methyl-B12) is successfully used for methylation. The drawbacks, however, are that it has a number of side effects and it has to be injected twice a week or daily. In addition, this medicine has not (yet) been approved in the Netherlands.

The importance of methylation has been satisfactorily demonstrated. It is still too early to claim that ascorbyl palmitate yields identical results as methyl-B12. While methyl-B12 can be used as a stand-alone therapy, I use ascorbyl palmitate only as part of my combined therapy.

Sometimes this combination of fat-soluble and water soluble Vitamin C without any other treatment gives very positive results, as the father of an autistic child recently informed me: '*Since our son began using the vitamin C his intellectual development has progressed considerably. At school he can function on a higher level, and he is even learning to read and write, which we at first believed to be impossible. We have become very enthusiastic about the use of vitamin C.*'

Instructive case with Lyme disease, application of detoxification in other diseases

It is not my intention to explain extensively here the homeopathic treatment of Lyme disease, but this case demonstrates how important *detoxification* is and that it can be used as a general principle in all kind of diseases. There is also another reason to show this case. After the detoxification, Vitamin C and fish oil were able to resolve the child's remaining problems which can be defined as oxidative stress in her brain.

Lyme disease is another disease that ravages the health of many people, and the frequency is still increasing. It can destroy health, render a person completely bedridden or even result in death. I have seen several cases and in my experience homeopathy is an excellent treatment for this disease. The magic formula is detoxification with the potentized disease itself. In fact, the same principle we use for the detoxification of vaccines, regular drugs or other diseases (e.g. mononucleosis) works for Lyme:

My patient was a 40-year-old woman whom I saw two years ago. She was infected with Lyme four years earlier. In the beginning she had a kind of influenza with severe headache and abdominal pain. She was sick for five weeks. Then she developed a severe neurological picture. She could hardly walk, the left part of her face became paralysed with her left eye half open and her bladder was difficult to empty because of weakness. Along with this she was exhausted and perspired profusely at night. She also became forgetful, which continued to the date of her visit. She had a perfusion with antibiotics over a three week period and had a thorough investigation to exclude Multiple Sclerosis. After the spinal tap she developed a high-pitched sound in her ears. Regardless of whether the course of antibiotics had ameliorated her general condition, she was not free from Lyme disease in an energetic sense. So two years later she worsened again and started a period of endless infections. The first was the most severe and dangerous, a pericarditis, followed by an inflammation of her optical nerve on the left side. This was followed by an infection of a left dental root and finally an acute bursitis of her left shoulder. A month before I saw her, she again had a severe relapse. It was clear that since the original infection she had suffered a long chain of health problems. She developed a severe headache, was hardly able to walk, was very stiff, even in her face and was completely exhausted. She requested new tests but her family doctor said that she had been treated correctly and if she wanted to go through all the medical investigations she had had before, it was her own choice.

Then I saw her. She was suffering from extreme weakness, headache, bad concentration and forgetfulness with difficult word-finding and pressure on her chest with restless sleep and palpitations.

I started the treatment with Lyme disease in homeopathic doses over eight weeks every potency, 30C through 10M, four times. In this way we go through the different levels of energy that are eventually infected. Here homeopathy shows clearly its power of subtle energetic intervention. After this course I saw her again and her first remark was: *'I feel great, Doc.'* Then she explained: *'I feel great after such a long time of constant misery. My energy is much better and I enjoyed pick- ing up my normal daily activities again. My headache has disappeared almost completely. Especially on the 200C I became nauseous and stiff in my face and on the 10M I had abdominal cramps and diarrhea. I am still forgetful and my concentration is not that good. The pain on my chest has improved a lot. My stool has completely changed, and I go to the bathroom every morning. I have completely stopped taking Paracetamol (a painkiller, which had been taken about four times a week). The beep in my head has not changed.'*

Then the homeopathic preparations of Lyme disease were repeated two more times to eradicate completely all traces of the disease left over the last six years. When the last course didn't give any further improvement, it was a clear sign to stop this treatment. One symptom that had appeared since she was infected with Lyme disease and did not disappear with the treatment was her forgetfulness and bad memory. Also the beep in her head caused by the lumbar puncture was still there. But remarkably, she was able to run without getting pain in her chest and her energy was excellent again.

We could have stopped her treatment here, but I like to go for 100% and so I started a more constitutional treatment with Cuprum 30C, which could also cure her Raynaud's. Five months later she was still excellent with a good energy, but the specific problems I was attempting to address had not disappeared. Cuprum 200C was not healing these specific problems either.

I reasoned that she still had a lot of stress, so-called oxidative stress, especially in her brain, due to her Lyme disease. Therefore, her concentration was bad and she still was very forgetful. So I prescribed ascorbyl palmitate 500mg three times a day, a complex of ascorbates three times a day and 1000mg fish oil a day as I have learned with autistic children. With that I also gave her 25mg zinc a day because she is a Cuprum personality (in the homeopathic analysis). For Cuprum type patients, zinc can lower copper levels and bring more relaxation.

At the end of almost five months she was enthusiastic again. She had believed that her state five months before was about the maximum level of health she could hope to attain, but now she was more alert and felt more relaxed and peaceful inside. But the most important improvement was her memory. Her forgetfulness was gone and her concentration was much better. Also the beep in her head had almost completely gone and most of the time she was not aware of it. She felt tremendous energy. During her holidays she had visited Barcelona with other people. A whole day touring about the streets in a big city is very exhausting for most people, but she was the only one of the group that still felt vigorous at the end of the day.

I tell this story, not only to show how nicely detoxification works, but also because it demonstrates that many complaints are linked with oxidative stress in the brain, as in autistic children, and that vitamin C is the pre-eminent remedy to heal this stress. Vitamin C deserves a much more important role in our health care than it actually has, and it can prevent many diseases that are due to stress. More importantly, it can heal the oxidative stress that is caused by different diseases or allopathic drugs. It now plays a prominent role in my treatment of autistic children.

The controversy over vitamin C

When I read the books and articles on vitamin C, and I started to prescribe relatively high doses of vitamin C myself in cancer patients and autistic children, it was surprising to discover that this vitamin has quite a bad reputation. Dr. Archie Kalokerinos from Australia, who saved so many Aboriginal children with the administration of vitamin C, was treated as a charlatan by some medical colleagues. Even the famous researcher Linus Pauling, who twice won the Nobel Prize for his research, was criticized because he promoted high doses of vitamin C. He died at 94 after using 13 grams of vitamin C himself every day for many years. Many doctors are startled when they hear about the high doses of vitamin C, far higher than what is normally admitted to be enough to avoid scurvy, i.e. 50-60mg a day.

However, the Western world has changed dramatically in the last fifty years. As a 60-year-old, I remember being born on a farm without running water, electricity, phone, TV or car. In winter we went to bed with an oil lamp and when it was freezing or there was a sharp frost, my mother passed an iron that was heated on the coal-fired stove through our bed. Just 50 years ago! We lived in nature and ate vegetables from our garden. In winter we ate cabbage and carrots and some preserves my mother made from fruits in and around our farm, instead of the exotic fruits and vegetables available nowadays.

We wore woolen or linen clothes and were well connected with Mother Earth by leather-soled or wooden shoes or even connected with our hands and feet when we were working on all fours in the field. The air was pure and our house was healthy, devoid of carpets full of chemicals, plastics and electronic equipment. I went to school on my bike through the beautiful countryside and when there was too much snow, we walked, enjoying the miracles of the pure, untouched landscape. While physically we might not have had such an easy life, mentally and emotionally there was much less stress. I can imagine that we had hardly any free radicals, and thus we needed no extra vitamin C to supplement the natural food high in vitamin C.

How different life is 50 years later. Everything has changed in the Western world. We suffer over-consumption, a thousand-fold increase in emotional stress and oxidative stress from pollution, decayed food and an unnatural environment. We have lost contact with the earth, wearing plastic or rubber shoes, and suffer from static electricity from our synthetic clothes and carpeting. Millions of children have only a polluted environment to play in with the risk of being killed by a car every minute. We pay the consequences of believing there is never enough and we need more and more. Buying the next new toy that comes on the market can only make us happy for a while until we again desire a bigger car or a bigger TV screen. We still cannot stop the massive delusion that having something will make us happier than we were before.

In this world our original need for vitamin C is quite insufficient. Human beings and guinea pigs are the only mammals that cannot produce their own vitamin C. We lack an enzyme to do so. Research has revealed that mice produce an amount of vitamin C equivalent 12 to 13 grams if translated our bodyweight. However, a goat under stress can produce up to a hundred grams (not milligrams!) per day. If all mammals produce high quantities of vitamin C to combat stress, how can we continue to believe that 60mg of vitamin C a day is enough for human beings, as the US government says in its Recommended Daily Allowances? Do we have another way to replace this deficiency? No!

There is still another argument that is mounted against high doses of vitamin C. It is claimed by some that our kidneys could be damaged by high doses of vitamin C or at least we might get kidney stones from it. Again no! If a goat, which has physiologically the same kidneys as human beings, does not get kidney stones, why should we? There is no medical proof or evidence that vitamin C can cause harm to our kidneys. In all these years I have never seen it happen; on the contrary, I saw so many wonderful results from high doses of vitamin C that for me there can be no doubt about its safety. Colleagues in the USA and Australia who have decades of experiences with high doses never saw this happen. Vitamin C is a most powerful remedy that even in very high doses, up to 80-90 grams by perfusion, does not give side effects. It has saved the lives of many children and adults. We should consider these assertions as superstition or ignorance. The only side effect that can be attributed to vitamin C is diarrhea, which is harmless and just means that you have to lower the quantity a little bit. (This is called the 'bowel tolerance test': you keep taking increased amounts of vitamin C until you get diarrhea, which indicates you have reached your upper limit.) The sicker the person is, the more he needs vitamin C and the higher the bowel tolerance dose becomes. Some other people suffer from acidity due to the ascorbic acid formula, because their digestive system is out of balance. That is why I generally use the ascorbate form, which is much better tolerated.

CHAPTER 7

FATTY ACIDS AND GLUTAMATES

Polyunsaturated fatty acids (omega-3 and omega-6 fatty acids) play a crucial role in the formation and functioning of the brain. The omega-3 fatty acid has been greatly reduced in our modern diet of processed food, while we get an overwhelming quantity of omega-6 fatty acids from the corn and soy added to processed foods.

Scientific research in recent years has revealed that an unsaturated fatty acid deficiency or an imbalance of unsaturated and saturated fatty acids may play an important role in behavioral disorders, learning problems, dyslexia and autistic spectrum disorders. Omega-3 fatty acids are found in fish, flaxseed oil (ALA), certain nuts and to a lesser extent in leafy greens. They are essential in the normal development of the brain as well as in our mental and emotional health. Pregnant women should take omega-3 supplements, and children under three years of age require large amounts of omega-3 fatty acids (EPA and DHA) for healthy brain development. Even after age three children should take sufficient fish oil to keep their brain in good condition and to make learning easier and more successful. I only prescribe the omega-3 fatty acids because omega-6 and omega-9 are already over represented in our food. The main problem is a lack of omega-3 fatty acids. The younger the children are the more they need DHA in relation to EPA, so especially during pregnancy and the first 3 years of life.

According to Dr. Alex Richardson from the UK, indications of an omega-3 fatty acid deficiency are:

1. Excessive thirst, frequent urination, rough or dry skin, dry lusterless hair, dandruff and soft brittle nails.

2. Allergic propensity: eczema, asthma, hay fever, etc.

3. Visual symptoms such as poor night vision, hypersensitivity to light and reading disorders such as dancing letters.

4. Attention disorders: quick distraction, poor concentration and memory disorders.

5. Emotional hypersensitivity: in particular tendencies to depression, intense mood swings and excessive fears.

6. Sleeping problems: in particular being unable to wind down at night and having difficulty waking up in the morning.

Vegetarian sources of omega-3 fatty acids such as flaxseed oil only contain ALA (alpha-linoleic acid) that is not always properly metabolized into EPA and DHA. For this reason direct supplementation of EPA/DHA in the form of fish oil is preferred. Research has shown that the ideal EPA intake for young children is about 500mg a day, but some people require even more.

DHA is especially important in the structure of brain cell membranes, particularly in early childhood when the brain grows and later on in life to retain flexibility of the membranes.

In children, 20% of the brain consists of DHA. EPA plays an essential part in the short-term regulation of brain functions such as hormonal balance, the immune function and the bloodstream. EPA is equally important in reducing infections, for instance in the digestive tract. Both fatty acids are indispensable for all cell membranes since they regulate the nourishment flow to the cell. They are also involved in the release and reabsorption of neurotransmitters (chemicals that are essential in stimulus transfer between neurons).

But there is still another important difference between omega-3 and omega-6 fatty acids. Omega-3 fatty acids are anti-inflammatory substances and help the immune system to prevent infections. Omega-6 fatty acids are pro-inflammatory substances that weaken the immune system and promote infections. That alone is reason enough to restore the balance between omega-3 and omega-6 fatty acids and to lower considerably the intake of omega-6 fatty acids with our food,

In ancient times the ratio between omega-3 and omega-6 fatty acids was about 1:1. This enabled our ancient ancestors, eating shellfish full of omega-3 fatty acids around Lake Victoria in Africa a million years ago, to develop their cortex and take the first steps towards becoming *homo sapiens*. Then some hundred thousand years ago these ancestors learned fishing and this again enabled the cortex to expand with all kinds of new possibilities: thinking, creativity, management of aggression, a fuller range of emotions and speech. This means without any doubt that we need omega-3 fatty acids to maintain our brain in good condition and to preserve our specific human qualities.

You do not have to be a scientist to appreciate the fact that our modern diet with a ratio of omega-3 to omega-6 of 1:20 or even 1:25 is jeopardizing our future as human beings. Even our most basic foods have changed. According to recent research, babies under one year of age in the US have doubled in fat because the milk they drink is delivered by cows that are fed with corn and soy beans containing omega-6 instead of omega-3 fatty acids provided by cows fed with grass. Omega-6 fatty acids stimulate the formation of fat. The fact that packaged food products contain on average 60% corn byproducts makes clear that the health of our body and especially of our brain has become dangerously dependent on a food industry that is only interested in making huge profits instead of providing healthy food to everybody.

Moreover, meat has changed drastically because our cattle are also fed with corn and soy, thereby lowering the omega-3 content of the meat and increasing the omega-6 fatty acids. The same is true for farmed fish because they are fed with corn and soy, in other words unnatural food for fish. Additionally, many products nowadays contain hydrogenated vegetable fats (hardened fats), for example margarine, mayonnaise, cookies, snacks, etc. All this insures that most people lack sufficient good fats (omega-3 fatty acids) to keep their brain and the rest of their body in good condition. Our body has no other choice than to use these fats as a replacement for the missing omega-3 fatty acids. In this way cell membranes and our brain become rigid.

Imagine a pregnant woman who is not especially aware of the dangers of our modern food system and is eating this degenerated food for 20 or 30 years. How can her baby develop a healthy body and especially a healthy brain? She cannot give to her baby what she does not have herself. Her baby will arrive in this world with a deficient and vulnerable brain. Just a few vaccines can be enough then to retard his healthy development and make him or her dependent on antibiotics, inhalers, cortisone ointments, Ritalin and the like.

Glutamate

And as if this is still not enough to make our health fragile and compromised, nearly all packaged food contains glutamates, the so-called MSG's (monosodium glutamates). MSG hides behind 25 or more names, such as Natural Flavoring, Accent, Aginomoto, Natural Meat Tenderizer, etc. In hundreds of studies around the world, scientists have created obese mice and rats by injecting them with MSG when they are first born to prepare them for use in diet or diabetes test studies. The MSG triples the amount of insulin the pancreas creates. John Erb, in his book *The Slow Poisoning of America,* says that MSG is added to food for the addictive effect it has on the human body; it just makes people eat more and become fat.

It is high time to stop all these poisonings in our daily diet and offer real food to our beloved children and to ourselves. Let us eat real food instead of edible products that do not deserve the name of food. Let us refuse to eat these denatured products that harm the health of our children and ourselves. There is only one solution to resolve this important issue: eat organic and fresh food, thereby making healthy food a central issue in our lifestyle.

In the next chapter I will talk about another poison that has invaded our food: sugar!

CHAPTER 8

INTESTINAL DISORDERS AND DIET

You would expect that in a multidisciplinary approach diet would play an important role, but I hardly ever prescribe a special diet. Why? Approximately 85% of autistic children experience intestinal and assimilation disorders. Should we not give probiotics and avoid food with gluten, dairy and the like to restore the intestinal balance again?

I am not opposed to these dietary interventions, but they are not truly curative, they create a great burden on the parents, and in most cases I have found them unnecessary. These food restrictions are a heavy burden for the parents and the burden is already very high. If the parents have already started with food restrictions before bringing their child to me, I always continue this. But if they haven't, I do not start food restrictions at the same time as my treatment, because this would make it hard to evaluate the results. Moreover, in most of my autistic patients the digestive system heals within some months without probiotics or changes in diet.

However, if the situation of the child is too dramatic, it is useful to start with a gluten, sugar and dairy-free diet, if possible after diagnostic tests. Sometimes it dramatically ameliorates the behavior of the child and makes all the struggle of food restrictions more than worth the effort.

Normally, the only guideline I ask the parents to follow is to give organic food without additives and to stop completely the use of added sweets, including artificial sweeteners. Most parents are not aware of the harmfulness of these substances. The addition of sweets is so common nowadays that it is accepted without question by most people. I consider sugar a very toxic substance to be avoided as much as possible. A very interesting book by Elaine Gottschall, *Breaking The Vicious Cycle* (2004), offers a deeper insight into what sugar does in our digestive system and what the consequences are for the entire physical system.

Around 1900 we used just one kilogram of added sugar per person per year. Today, we use an average of 70 kilograms per person per year. Since some people avoid sugar, many people must be using far higher doses. This is absolutely toxic and gives a lot of oxidative stress. Autistic children and children with behavioral problems (ADHD, aggressive children, etc.) in general should therefore be put on a sugar-free diet. It goes together with my treatment with Saccharum officinale, which is also made from sugar (the juice of sugar cane), following the principle of using a homeopathic remedy made from a toxic substance to cure problems caused by that substance.

Elaine Gottschall explains how disaccharides and polysaccharides (complex sugars) are responsible for a lot of trouble in our digestive system. The only sugar that the body can digest is glucose. Therefore all sugars that enter into our body have to be transformed first into glucose. This process is only possible with enzymes that are produced by the body itself.

Unlike sucrose, lactose and starch, glucose does not need any digestion and therefore is readily absorbed in the small intestines. Disaccharides, such as beet and cane sugar (sucrose), as well as lactose, (iso)maltose and polysaccharides cannot be absorbed in the small intestines and enter the colon where they nourish 'sugar-addicted' bacteria, which in their turn disturb, by their proliferation, the balance of useful and necessary bacteria of the digestive system. These sugar-eating bacteria enter the small intestines en masse and cause irritable bowels, which produce mucus as a protection, and diarrhea. The disaccharides make no contact with the absorbing cells of the colon and are food for the sugar-eating bacteria. These bacteria produce toxins that are absorbed into the blood and enter the brain, causing oxidative stress and behavior problems. Sugar and other sweets also stimulate the growth of Candida albicans in the bowels, a yeast responsible for a wide range of complaints. Through the malabsorption of vitamins and minerals the brain can become dysfunctional, setting the stage for epilepsy, confusion, aggression, disorientation, poor judgment, strange and bizarre behavior, speech problems, unsteady gait, loss of memory, etc. While this connection may seem farfetched, we find that simply eliminating all sugars from the diet can sometimes reverse this long list of problems.

Normally, the stomach and the upper part of the small intestine contain very few bacteria. Overgrowth of bacteria in the stomach and upper part of the small intestine can produce a wide variety of health problems including malabsorption of nutrients due to destruction of important enzymes. Lactase is one of the first enzymes that are damaged. That is why so many children (and adults) have problems with milk and milk products. These digestive problems can be tackled with the Specific Carbohydrate Diet that deprives these wrong bacteria of their food and restores the enzymes necessary for good digestion. The problem with this diet is not so much its efficacy but the difficulties in following it (you even have to bake your own bread) and its blandness.

The Metallothionein Story

The story of the protein metallothionein can help us to understand how intestinal problems can persist and how this affects brain function at the same time. Metallothionein is our first line of defense against heavy metals. It is present in the mouth, stomach and in large quantities in the intestines. If sufficient metallothionein is present in the intestine, heavy metals such as mercury, aluminum or lead will be bound to this protein by the exchange of zinc. Enzymes that break down casein and gluten also need zinc for their functioning. Therefore, a metallothionein deficiency will lead to a deficiency of the enzyme that breaks down casein and gluten. This in turn leads to a casein and gluten allergy. If the metallothionein protein is not functioning because of lack of zinc it causes mercury, lead and other heavy metals to end up in the blood. According to Dr. William J. Walsh, Ph.D., biochemical researcher at the Pfeiffer Treatment Center, the malfunctioning of this protein in the mouth may lead to taste disorders and eating problems so often seen in autistic children. Very often they refuse to eat solid food with lumps or have strange food behaviors, refusing most foods and focusing on only a few.

Metallothionein also protects against infection of the intestine and can heal the diarrhea so common among autistic children. Even Candida and other fungi may be tackled by this protein.

Heavy metals are very toxic for the human body, especially for the brain, which is why metallothionein plays such an important role in the first line defense of our digestive system. In a greatly polluted world it is essential for our health and even our survival. The daily intake of mercury from food is about 20mcg; if teeth are filled with amalgam, an extra dose is added depending on the age of the amalgam (1mcg/day for old amalgam to 450mcg/day for new amalgam) according to the Pfeiffer Institute. We also ingest heavy metals with the air we breathe. Fortunately metallothionein is also present to protect our body.

The problem with heavy metals in vaccines is that it bypasses the defense lines of our body and infects our blood directly. Aluminum is also present in all kinds of packaging materials; juice packs are typically lined with aluminum. Many people still cook using aluminum pots, especially when on holiday. The brain cannot protect itself completely against the entrance of heavy metals notwithstanding the blood-brain barrier, therefore metallothionein is a really essential protein. No wonder that a history of millions of years of adjustment to our environment has also provided us with metallothionein in the brain. But if it is functioning at a low level because of zinc deficiency, which almost all autistic children seem to have, there is a dangerous situation of intoxication. These children are extremely sensitive to their environment and need to get organic and fresh food, avoiding all packaging with heavy metals in it.

Research by Dr. William J. Walsh, Ph.D., biochemical researcher of the Pfeiffer Treatment Center, Illinois found that when he tested more than 500 autistic children, they all had an abnormally high level of unbound copper in the blood.

Metallothionein is an important supplier of zinc to the cell and in particular to the white blood cells (leucocytes) which are of vital importance for our immune system. With a zinc deficiency an early shift from cellular to humeral defense takes place which leads to immunological decline. Vaccines also provoke the same shift from cellular to humeral defense. Zinc deficiency in children may also lead to growth disorders and impaired development of genital and endocrine function.

According to the Pfeiffer Institute, a poorly functioning metallothionein system also explains why boys are 4 times more likely than girls to develop autism. Girls are better protected against external toxic materials because estrogen and progesterone (female hormones) stimulate metallothionein production.

An important cause of zinc deficiency may be the consumption of whole-wheat yeast bread. This type of bread contains phytic acid that forms an insoluble complex with zinc and thus blocks zinc assimilation. The solution to this is sourdough bread since sourdough dissolves phytic acid.

CHAPTER 9

AGGRESSIVENESS

Many parents of autistic children are confronted with the aggressive behavior of their child, which makes the whole situation even more difficult. I once saw in my office an eleven-year-old autistic child who needed four adults to restrain him. He was biting, kicking and hitting not only himself but also whoever he could reach. In many cases the parents have to separate their autistic child from their siblings, and often mothers are threatened and hit or bitten by their child. Why are so many autistic children aggressive?

Aggression is part of our old brain, the limbic system. Aggressive behavior in animals, which is part of their survival instinct, is located there as well. In human beings this aggressiveness is controlled by the neocortex, which is the largest and most recently developed part of our brain. Without this control we would not be able to behave as human beings. The development of the neocortex has transformed our primitive ancestors of a million years ago to the human being of today, able to think, to be creative, to talk, to have all kind of emotions, to express love, to walk upright and to execute complicated movements like piano playing. From this point of view the question can be raised if killing each other (not only murder but also government-sanctioned killings as in war and executions) is part of a normally-functioning human brain endowed with a wonderful organ called the neocortex. Or how is it possible that human beings can be so uncontrolled that they rape, commit incest, fight with each other, or be so angry that they commit the most horrible injuries to their fellow human beings, or steal from others, or gather billions of money just for their own benefit while their neighbors are starving?

Is this part of a healthy functioning human brain or should such a behavior be considered pathological?

I fully agree with Eckhart Tolle who says in *The Power of Now* and *A New Earth*, that humanity is severely ill. If so, shouldn't we approach these problems completely differently? Shouldn't we stop just putting people in jail without any treatment as if criminality is just their free choice? Shouldn't we stop also punishing our children when they behave unacceptably and instead try to heal their brain? Shouldn't we try to find out what is wrong with a child rather than forcing him to do what we want? I hear you thinking: "But there is no such treatment available". You just can go to a psychologist when the problems become too severe and he will treat the child with behavioral therapy which is mostly not very effective. Or if the problems are severe enough you can go to a psychiatrist who will put your child on Ritalin, Concerta, or even on Haloperidol (Haldol, an antipsychotic drug). In any case the child will not heal from his disease and become once more a healthy, well-behaved child. At best, his problems will be more manageable. No, we need a more subtle approach able to restore the normal control function of the neocortex. Does such an approach exist then? Yes, homeopathy has the tools to heal these children on a deep level without using any poison and without making them dependant on toxic drugs. I will give an example.

A case of an aggressive child cured with classical homeopathy

Pauline is just at the brink of puberty, thirteen years old. Everything goes to extremes in her life. She has extreme mood swings, excessive joy alternating with extreme anger and aggressiveness. She is unable to get over minor frustrations and she completely loses her control, whether in the presence of friends or strangers. For the whole family it is a disaster and it is almost impossible to get her out of her cranky mood. She always has a strong negative attitude. She is rather introverted and has a strong fear of failure. Curiously she mostly is extremely happy and active after dinner, but the smallest incident can precipitate her into the abyss of furor. She is unpredictable and dislikes changes. She terrorizes the whole family with her behavior, while at school she is timid and well behaved.

These contradictory moods and behavior, as if the person has two different personalities, are a keynote for the homeopathic remedy Anacardium orientale. So she was prescribed this remedy in a 30C potency, once a week. I saw her for follow-up three months later.

At her first dose she already had a strong reaction. She had abdominal pain and after three days she became dizzy and fainted.

In the second week she started to improve. She was calmer, more in control, and her extreme fits of anger disappeared although she was still angry frequently. Then in the third week she was rather depressed and withdrawn, she locked herself up in her bedroom and felt sorry for herself. She stayed for three weeks in this state.

Then her mood changed completely and she became lovable, pleasant, social, affectionate and enjoying life. She again phoned her friends and made plans to see them. She was a pleasure to be around, or as her mother said: "My old Pauline is back again".

The question is how can a subtle, purely energetic homeopathic intervention heal this girl so profoundly? Not an easy question to answer. First we have to establish the fact that it does. These healings with homeopathy are not exceptional. The first step in understanding her healing is to understand what is wrong in the functioning of this young girl. Why isn't her neocortex doing its job: to control her basic emotions? This is important to understand why autistic children are so often aggressive or have other uncontrolled behaviors. I earlier stated that the brains of autistic children are not damaged but blocked. Blocked or dysfunctional brains have no physical lesion but have functional disturbances, corresponding to an energetic unbalance.

This dysfunction can even be provoked by a substance that is no longer present. Suppose the brain is poisoned with mercury. The mercury provokes an imprint on the energetic functioning of the brain. Then the mercury is taken out by chelation therapy, but the imprint stays unchanged and continues to block the normal functioning of the brain. Not chelation therapy but homeopathy can erase these imprints and restore the normal functioning of the brain. That is why homeopathy is so effective in the treatment of behavioral problems.

In this example it is easy to understand that punishment will not help either the girl nor the parents. Pauline is also very unhappy with the whole situation, but is overpowered by her dysfunctional brain. I am convinced that many unfortunate juvenile delinquents could become peaceful adolescents again with appropriate treatment. Jailing them for years, then releasing them with the same dysfunctional brain pattern is a setup for relapse. We have to heal them instead of putting them in jail. With homeopathy we can remove the wrong imprints in the brains.

Recent research on the memory of water has also shown that imprints can stay for an indefinite time. Months after water had been completely chemically purified from mercury contamination, this same water still showed the imprints of mercury by spectrographic resonance. (Dr. Prof. Herbert Klima of the Atomic Institute of Vienna in Austria)

I noticed years ago that many children with post-vaccination syndrome had aggressive behavior which disappeared completely when the vaccines were detoxified systematically. It is my strong conviction that one of the main reasons for the increase of aggressiveness in our modern world is the increase in vaccinations. But which part of the vaccine is responsible? Vaccines contain mercury or aluminum, both being neurotoxins. Both metals are well known as homeopathic remedies described in our materia medica. When we look at the symptoms associated with the homeopathic remedy Mercury, aggression is a striking part of the picture. It is present in the rubric (symptom) 'desire to kill' in the third degree, which means that this symptom has been observed frequently and has been confirmed clinically. But this is not all. This metal is also present in rubrics such as: 'anger that he could have stabbed any one'; insanity; rage, fury and violence. If we look at the remedy Aluminum, we find a picture that is less aggressive (apart from the symptom 'desire to kill at the sight of a knife or gun'). However, we find symptoms such as absent minded, anxiety, fear, indolence, imbecility, insanity, prostration of mind, and depression, a picture that is not very joyful either.

To make a killer out of a child without being caught and put in jail for many years, one would only need to inject very small quantities of mercury at regular intervals starting at birth. In this way the child will become a 'Mercury child' with all the tendencies of a Mercury personality as outlined above. If you want a child to become stubborn, insane, depressed, and unable to use his brain to its full extent, just do the same thing with aluminum oxide or aluminum hydroxide — in other words, just what we are doing with vaccinations. And what will happen if we regularly inject very small quantities of formaldehyde into our newborns?

Nevertheless this is what we are doing to our little children worldwide. Can we really be surprised that aggression is increasing in our society while intelligence in many of our children is decreasing? I anticipate the objection that if these vaccines were not safe they would immediately be stopped, that they are proven safe by scientific research. Alas, I have to disappoint you. There is simply no good research which compares vaccinated children with unvaccinated children. The existing research compares children who have had one vaccine with children who have had a different one — but both groups of children have had the same additives such as mercury, aluminum, formaldehyde and other additives.

There is to my knowledge only one way to get these toxins and their imprints out of the brains of our children and that is the detoxification of vaccines with homeopathic preparations of these very vaccines. Then we have to reconsider the worldwide practice of vaccination and look for better solutions to keep our children healthy and to avoid major catastrophes of contagious diseases. Here the homeopathic version of vaccinations, which are completely safe and without side-effects could play an important role. For more information the interested reader should read the book of Dr. Isaac Golden, *Vaccination & Homeoprophylaxis, A Review of Risks and Alternatives*; 6th edition, ISBN 978-0-9578726-4-6. We should much more think in terms of decreasing vaccinations rather than to increase them. We should also reconsider the very early vaccination of our children and rather protect their health in a more natural way, at least the first two years without any vaccination when their brains are still so vulnerable. I will come back to this last statement later in this chapter when discussing the Japanese experience in the seventies and eighties. Let us first give some examples how the fragile brains of our children are intoxicated by vaccines. Homeopathy has the tools to prove the connection between their suffering and the vaccinations they received. The following cases have been published already in an international homeopathic journal, *The Homeopathic Links*. In this article the focus was not specifically on aggressiveness but on behavioral problems in general.

Eight cases of behavioral problems strongly improved by detoxification
Ross (3 years) got epilepsy after the MMR and also became very restless and aggressive. After two courses of potentized MMR he becomes much happier, calmer and his aggressiveness disappeared completely. He is not hitting other children and himself any more. He can play alone now and can sit still at the table during his meals.

Amy (3½ years) had a severe convulsion with unconsciousness lasting three hours, 16 days after the MMR shot. Then she gradually developed epilepsy which was treated with Depakine. Her mood changed completely after that shot. She became very aggressive, angry and unmanageable. Often she was tired; after getting up in the morning she would lie down on the couch. After the potentized MMR her energy and her behavior become normal again. Her aggressiveness and anger are now completely gone and she is happy and open again, 'the old Amy.' And what is more, the epilepsy disappeared gradually as well and she is now free of complaints without Depakine. Like many others, the case was not recognised by the authorities as post-vaccination damage.

Fleur (18 months) started to be very aggressive after her fourth DTPP/Hib at 11 months, and her motor development was slowing down. She even hit her physiotherapist. She also had four ear infections. After the MMR shot her aggressiveness became even worse. Three courses of potentized MMR and three of DTPP/Hib changed her completely. Her aggressiveness disappeared, the sweating on her head stopped, her stool became solid and her speech progressed again.

Rik (4 years): diagnosis autism. He had been a perfectly normal child until the MMR vaccination at 16 months. He had developed rapidly, had been able to go up and down the stairs by himself. In the first week after his MMR shot he regressed rapidly, mentally as well as physically. His behavior changed dramatically: he became aggressive, was uncontrollable at the daycare center, made screeching noises, withdrew from strangers, his speech completely disappeared and his physical development stopped and even regressed. He became a poor sleeper. Eye contact was no longer possible. His pupils were fully contracted and no longer responded to light. There was no way to correct him. He had soft stools and frequent nosebleeds.

After five courses of potentized MMR much was accomplished. His pupils reacted to light again and eye contact was reestablished. The nosebleeds stopped and he slept well again. He resumed speaking and formed two or three word sentences. He was once again aware of and responsive to his environment, for instance at one point he suddenly became afraid of seeing a mother duck with ducklings whereas before he never had shown any response to such a scene. He was able to reach out and make contact. He hugged his parents and people he loved. He comforted his sister when she cried. His restlessness was gone and he was able to follow instructions. His fears decreased and his self-mutilating tendencies completely disappeared along with his aggressiveness. During each potentized MMR series he screamed just as he had when he received the original MMR vaccination, but afterwards he steadily improved. He was back to being a normal child. The veils had been lifted.

Joep (2 years) was a nice child without problems until four or five months after the MMR. Then his behavior changed completely. He became very aggressive, easily angered, knocking his head on the floor and hitting other children and himself. The whole family was upset by his behavior. He was sent to a psychotherapist by the pediatrician when he was 2 years and 3 months old! After one course of potentized MMR his behavior became completely normal again, he stopped hitting himself and other children, and the head-banging ceased right away. He relapsed many times about 2 weeks after the MMR course, but again and again his behavior became normal after the potentized MMR. Finally after many repetitions of the homeopathic MMR he remained the joyful and nice child he was before.

Jeroen is diagnosed ADHD-PDD-NOS. This sixteen-year-old became depressed after the MMR and DTPol shot at 9 years. Before he was a calm and well-behaved boy, without any problems at school, but after these double shots he didn't want to go to school, complaining of headaches and abdominal pains. He became aggressive, awkward and uncertain in his contact with other children. He was tired, had no day-night rhythm anymore, and played truant by shutting himself in his bedroom and barricading the door. He had never displayed this odd behavior before. Once he became a teenager, he did what he wanted and refused any parental control. He was very restless and had difficulty falling asleep. Often he was absent-minded, inaccessible and easily irritated. He was on Ritalin, which made his behavior at school more acceptable, but his concentration was still a major problem.

After treatment with potentized DTPol and MMR his normal behavior and peaceful inner state came back again, especially with the potentized MMR. He could discontinue Ritalin without any problem, his concentration became normal, and his aggressive behavior disappeared as snow under the sun.

Nick, age two and a half, was diagnosed as probable ADHD. He was very restless, unmanageable, very aggressive toward other children, hitting, kicking, punching and shoving them. For the first three months of his life he cried continuously, and real contact was hardly possible. In his mother's womb he was already restless, causing his mother two bruised ribs. At the time of the first consult he was pale, very open, talking continuously, touching everything, unable to concentrate and with unrestrained outbursts of anger. He refused to form emotional bonds from the very beginning and never sat on his mother's lap. He had a tendency to infections and had already had eight rounds of antibiotics. His repetitive ear infections started at four months, and at one and a half his adenoids were removed. Both parents had tropical vaccinations 4 years before his mother got pregnant, including DTP, yellow fever and hepatitis A, which explains the early onset of his problems before his vaccinations started at two months. After every vaccination he reacted with a high fever. Two days after the MMR he got an acute inflammation of his hip joints, which was rapidly tackled with antibiotics. The homeopathic treatment was started with MMR, three courses, but without any change. Then DTPP/Hib, given in ascending potencies, changed him completely. He had a strong urticaria-like skin reaction, and a very foul and acrid loose stool, which are both detox reactions. Then his aggressiveness disappeared almost completely. Now he is much calmer, is happy and gentle and sits on his mother's lap to kiss her and to cuddle as he never did before. He is relaxed and not hyperactive any more. He is a completely different child, his mother says.

Tom (6 years); diagnosed with ADHD. All his problems started immediately after the MMR at 14 months. He passed out for five minutes, and about two hours later he got a urticaria (nettle rash) reaction all over his body lasting one day. After that he was a completely different child. Before he was quiet, then he became restless, disobedient and destructive. Before he had a good appetite eating almost everything, afterwards he had poor appetite and was a fussy eater. Before he slept until 7 a.m., afterwards he woke at 5 a.m. At school he was still well-behaved, but at home he would turn away from his mother, tap with sticks on everything, and throw stones and sand at other children. He had frequent fits of anger, he kicked and hit even his mother and he was insolent. Without any reason he would hit other children in the stomach. His concentration was poor, and he played purposelessly. He would sweat a lot during the night. His stool was loose and very foul.

During the first course of potentized MMR extended over 2 months, he behaved like a one year old baby, sitting on the lap of his mother and sucking his thumb. He became much calmer, played normally again, was approachable and not aggressive anymore. He would sleep until 7 a.m again. He became again 'my little boy like before', says the mother. From time to time his behavior becomes a 'mess' again, he becomes touchy and reacts to everything. Then he himself asks for his little pills of potentized MMR, which again make him a calm and affectionate child for weeks or months.

Homeopathy using Isotherapy or a classical remedy can transform these disabled children again into healthy children with healthy brain function. We can ask why these vaccination side-effects are almost never diagnosed by pediatricians, neurologists and family doctors. First of all there are hardly comparisons anymore, because virtually all children are vaccinated. Therefore many complaints of our little children are considered to be normal and part of their development. Repeated ear infections, chronic runny noses, bronchitis, eczema, digestive problems and the many behavioral problems children have are classified as part of their normal development without any awareness within the medical profession that these complaints are not normal and are caused by vaccination or other medications. Children are vaccinated also from their first days or months of life, so that parents don't know what their little child would have been like without these medical interventions.

To make vaccination acceptable to the general public, it was also necessary to make doctors and parents believe that vaccines have no side-effects and are one of the most beautiful inventions of our modern medicine. The belief is so strong nowadays that every attempt to question vaccination is considered as an act of stupidity or malevolence. And then we have the enormous propaganda of the pharmaceutical industry itself. I will not go into details here but whoever wants to know how this works, should search the internet on the introduction of the new vaccine against cervical cancer. Without any scientific proof that this vaccine is safe or effective, it has been introduced in the US, in Holland and many other countries by people who have financial interest in the pharmaceutical industry which is producing it. Enormous campaigns have convinced the governments, official institutes responsible for the execution of this vaccination program and the population that this will be one more blessing for humanity. But this vaccine has already turned out to be harmful; girls have died or become paralyzed from it in the US.

Because powerful institutions like the pharmaceutical industry, the medical establishment and the government are so heavily involved with vaccinations and other drugs, the real causes of autism will not easily come to light for the next ten or twenty years. The only way to get scientific evidence is to organise independent comparative research between vaccinated and unvaccinated children. But this kind of research is carefully avoided because the outcome could be too far-reaching and create doubts about vaccinations.

Another problem is that conventional medicine has no diagnostic tools to verify whether vaccinations are involved in children's health problems. Most pediatricians and family doctors prefer to deny vaccination damage vigorously so as not to endanger their own reputation. They have no time to study the whole vaccination issue in depth — it is too complex and difficult to understand. The pharmaceutical industry has long since understood this and is the main provider of information to the medical world, not just for vaccinations, but for all medical information. The whole cholesterol affair is another excellent example of how doctors and the entire medical world has become victim of successful pharmaceutical promotion activities.

One of the most successful changes modern medicine could do, in order to stop the plague of autism and many other behavioral and health problems in our children, would be to postpone vaccination until the age of two. But then, wouldn't our children be exposed to all kinds of dangerous diseases successfully combated by early vaccination? To answer this important question we can look at Japan's experience in the 1970s (*Paediatrics* Volume 81 no 6 part 2; Report of the Task Force on Pertussis and Pertussis Immunization-1998). In 1975 Japan started the pertussis vaccination (included in the DPT vaccine) at 24 months instead of 3 months of age. In the preceding 5-year period, from 1970 until 1974, vaccination of pertussis was still done at 3 months and serves as comparison period. In the early period there had been 57 declared severe neurological reactions reported (encephalitis, convulsions, sudden death, infantile spasms) with sequelae and with 37 deaths. In the following 5 years from 1970 to 1974, with the pertussis vaccination (DPT) being given at 2 years, the severe side-effects dropped to 8 with only 3 deaths. In the 5 year period from 1981 to 1984 the number of severe neurological side-effects dropped even further to 5 with only 2 deaths. Also the neurological side-effects without sequelae dropped in these three periods from 82 to 34 and finally to 14. The writers conclude: *'Thus, the age of starting routine immunization appears to be a far more important determinant of temporally associated reactions than the switch from conventional whole-cell vaccines to acellular vaccines.'*

In Japan early vaccination was reintroduced because of an increase in pertussis. But the whole pertussis problem has been created by the immunization itself. Without vaccination a mother transmits her own antibodies against whooping cough to her baby who will be protected in the first year of his life. This is just the time that whooping cough can cause death. Now babies have no effective antibodies against this disease because their mothers were vaccinated. Before vaccination, whooping cough could be a terrible disease (unless treated homeopathically) but few children died from it. In Holland we have had regular epidemics since 1995 with thousands of cases because the vaccine is still made from a stem dating from the sixties (as everywhere in the world) and the bacteria has mutated since that time. The claim that vaccinated children would have less severe symptoms is yet another way to mislead the general public – especially considering that more than 90% of children who get whooping cough in Holland actually have been vaccinated against it.

Critics may say that even if we could postpone vaccinations until age two in the Western world without an increased risk for our little children, what about developing countries? Many thousands of children still die from measles, and tuberculosis is still ravaging children and adults. And in some countries babies still die from tetanus. Can vaccinations also be postponed in developing countries? Before answering, let us go to research published in 2000 but kept silent ever since.

This research comparing vaccinated children with unvaccinated children (the only real effective and true research concerning vaccination damage) in Guinea-Buissau finds that early vaccination is harmful to babies. In the *British Medical Journal* of 2000;321:1435 Kristensen, Aaby and Jensen published a study entitled *Routine vaccinations and child survival: follow up study in Guinea-Bissau, West Africa.* This research was methodologically correct and was published with the full agreement of the WHO. They found that children under one year of age had an almost double mortality rate if they were vaccinated with the DTPol vaccine than unvaccinated children of the same age.

How can these results be explained? The main problem in developing countries is hygiene; without hygiene vaccinations are hardly effective. Vaccines lower the effectiveness of the immune system and in a world with bad hygiene, children are more at risk from a weakened immune system than from the diseases prevented by vaccines. It was proved by extended research by the WHO itself that the BCG (Bacil Calmette-Guérin for tuberculosis) vaccination in India in the 1970s had no effect at all. The conclusion of this 7½ year research study in Madras, South India was: *'The distribution of new cases of bacillary tuberculosis among those not infected at intake did not show any evidence of a protective effect of the BCG vaccines.'* (*Bulletin of the World Health Organisation* 57 (5): 819-827 (1979). 260,000 people were involved in this study, which is the biggest research ever done with the BCG vaccine. But worldwide vaccine policy with such an ineffective vaccine has not changed since. Despite virtually all children in these countries with bad hygiene being vaccinated from their first day of existence, tuberculosis is still a huge health hazard affecting millions of people. How can a BCG protect if the real tuberculosis is not protecting those who had the illness earlier in their life? The Netherlands, which has never had systematic vaccination for tuberculosis, has had and maybe still has the lowest incidence of tuberculosis in the world for many years — a fact that needs serious reflection.

My heart turns upside down when I see advertisements by a major children's organization promoting vaccination of pregnant women to prevent tetanus in newborns. This tetanus problem only occurs in countries with bad hygiene, where the umbilical cord is cut with infected, dirty knives or bamboo, or the stump is rubbed with cow dung. But first, there is no scientific evidence that the tetanus vaccine is effective, and second, vaccination during pregnancy leads to high health risks. These vaccinations will not resolve the problem at all. Why not invest Western money in the education of professional midwifes who are aware of the real problem and who improve the hygiene during pregnancy, birth and infancy?

When I was in Nepal in September 2008 for our homeopathic project, supporting the education of Homeopathic Health Assistants (descriped at the end of this book) and preparing the education of homeopathic doctors at university level (BHMS), I visited with Rabindra Puri, our representative and executive director, in a small village where he has built a school for the local people. He showed me a child of about 6 years, who was the son of one of the teachers and who was the terror of the whole village. The next day I saw him at the Bhaktapur Homeopathic Clinic where I was doing supervision. After thorough investigation it became clear that the double tetanus vaccination during his mother's pregnancy was probably responsible for his autism. So I started to detoxify this tetanus vaccine and the results were spectacular. Within a few weeks his behavior changed completely and he became an almost normal child again. The whole village was amazed to see such a tremendous change in this boy whom everybody knew as an odd child. Now half of the village is descending to the Kathmandu Valley for homeopathic treatment.

It is clear that the brains of our children, especially before the age of two, are very vulnerable and deserve full protection instead of repeated attacks by our multiple vaccinations. The whole system of vaccination deserves a serious revision and correct scientific research independent of the pharmaceutical industry.

Dr. Thomas Jefferson, board member of the European Program for Improved Vaccination Safety Surveillance and head of the division of the Cochrane Collaboration, has announced that most safety studies on childhood vaccines are useless. *'There is some good research, but it is overwhelmed by the bad'*, he has stated. *'The public has been let down because proper studies have not been done.'*

(Source: Telegraph UK, *Vaccines expert warns studies are useless*, by Lorraine Fraser, Media Correspondent (Filed: 27/10/2002) http://consumercide.com/health/vacc-jefferson01.html)

I will not finish this chapter without giving two examples of aggressiveness in an autistic adolescent and in an adult. In fact aggressiveness is not a great problem in the healing process of these patients. Mostly their aggressiveness disappears without any problem, by detoxifying the same causes that have also generated the autism itself.

Aggressiveness in a adolescent

Luuk was eleven years old when he came to my office for the first time with his mother. He had been diagnosed recently as PDD-NOS. He had severe behavior problems; especially his aggressiveness and his incorrigibility made the family situation very hard for his mother who had to bring up her son alone. The father had suddenly left the family announcing that he had another girlfriend. Since then the behavior of Luuk strongly deteriorated, but in fact the problems had already started when he was six months old. At birth he was a perfect child, developed without any problem, had a bright and open expression and radiated a great satisfaction. But at six months he became restless, started to sleep badly, stayed wide awake and cried frequently. It did not even help for his mother to take him into her own bed; she had to keep him awake until he was exhausted hoping that he would sleep then for some hours. This demanding situation lasted until he was 18 months old. His speech did not develop until he was two and a half, and there was no eye-contact. His whole physical and emotional development was delayed. He needed full attention and his presence was overwhelming.

When he was five, he became unmanageable at home. He was hot-tempered, stamping his feet with anger, shrieking, slamming doors and throwing his toys around. His general development showed an increasing gap with his peer group. The family doctor did not support his mother at all, stating that it was her fault for being unable to handle her son. When he was eight the situation at school became unbearable. He was unable to follow normal schooling and was placed in a special school for children with behavior problems and developmental delays. At that time he was very irritable, extremely obstinate and hard to handle. He would beat up his sister and mother; his father had just left home once and for all.

So far no doctor made a correct diagnosis and nobody blamed the vaccinations he received so early in his life. So at nine years he got without any hesitation the booster shots of MMR and DTPol. The main change then was his loss of energy. He could not do anything and after school he would just lie down on the couch.

At the first consultation it is not difficult to retrace the whole story and to conclude that he has a severe post-vaccination syndrome. I decide to detox all his vaccines. Along with that he was given fish oil, 500mg per day, and Saccharum 30C once a week.

After 10 weeks there are already big improvements, just with the detox of DTPol and MMR. The DTPol made him quiet again and restored his sound sleep with a natural feeling of tiredness. His food allergies also considerably diminished. His perception of cold and warm also became normal. Before he just put on a t-shirt in winter. The reactions on the MMR detoxification were quite strong in the beginning. He became extremely angry and aggressive and threatened to cut his veins with a knife. The improvement on the DTPol detox seemed completely lost. But before long he improved again and even became compliant. He felt relaxed as never before and said that he did not need to restrain himself anymore. 'This is Luuk as I knew him as a baby', exclaimed his mother.

Then the DTPP and Hib were detoxified, which brought more and more improvement. He was able to sense the feelings of others and was not stuck so long in negative moods anymore. The tired feeling in his head was gone also, and his concentration slowly improved. His activities increased again. Then the treatment was continued with the higher potencies of Saccharum, and almost two years after the start of his treatment his mother evaluated his overall healing at 80%. So far the detoxification of his vaccines reached the expected success, so that Inspiring Homeopathy could be applied successfully to get 100% healing.

Then I switch the homeopathic treatment to Hydrogenium 30C once a week. Hydrogenium has this wonderful capacity to connect people again with their essence, the person they really are. Because Luuk had lost his identity through all these vaccinations, I chose this remedy. This remedy has completely restored his balance and has healed the remaining 20% of his symptoms. He is much calmer and happier and he is performing well at school. And even his relationship with his father, which had been bad since he left home, has substantially improved. A long story of suffering for him and his family, especially his mother, has finally come to an end. At this stage his mother uses for the first time the word 'fantastic' to describe her son's healing.

Case of aggressiveness in a young adult

David was 18 years old when his parents brought him to my office for the first time. They had tried already many treatments. His first diagnosis when he was one year old was mental retardation. At five years the diagnosis was adjusted to autistic-like behavior and at age seventeen as autism. His problems started in a very early stage of his life. He was not reacting properly to different stimuli, although a hearing test did not reveal anything wrong. He walked at 32 months and was potty trained at six and a half. His speech developed very slowly with frequent echolalia (a kind of automatic repetition typical of autism). Even nowadays he only uses single words or short sentences. His comprehension is limited. He has obsessive behavior, turning around a ball or staring for hours at the turning drum of a washing machine. He is not able to play by himself and always needs somebody. The eye-contact is good as if his eyes are expressing more than he can physically perform.

His mother had severe diabetes during her pregnancy and was hospitalized. Apart from that her pregnancy was uneventful and I did not find any other causative factor in his medical history except the vaccinations for the early onset of his autism and for his retardation. He received the standard vaccinations, and at age fifteen he was given a vaccination against meningitis C (Neisvac-C) after which he had a high fever and was extremely tired. Then his previously nice character changed profoundly. He became cross and aggressive, pushing and hitting other people and his parents. He did not obey anymore and became almost impossible for his parents to handle. He wanted to sleep all the time, and physical exercise became too exhausting. After a year the situation slowly improved, only to deteriorate again two years later without apparent reason. He was very attached to his mother, wanted to hold her hand all the time and hardly allowed her to move. Again his aggressiveness increased with spitting, shrieking and hitting. He was very difficult to handle.

I preferred to treat first his meningococcal vaccination as it had such a bad effect on him and made him aggressive. Along with that he received ascorbyl palmitate 500mg twice a day, glutathione 75mg twice a day and fish oil 1000mg once a day. I also prescribed also Saccharum LM6 twice a week.

Within six weeks, after the detox of his meningococcal vaccine, his aggressiveness was completely gone. No spitting, no shrieking, no hitting anymore at home and at school. He was calmer and more relaxed, and his weakness disappeared slowly. He could be taken for a walk again.

Then his Havrix vaccination (hepatitis A and B) were detoxified, then the MMR, then the DTPP.

After a year of treatment much has been achieved already. Although his parents and his school feel he is still too passive and is not yet performing up to his potential, his aggressiveness is definitely gone. Further treatment should bring even more improvement.

CHAPTER 10

COMPLETE AND ALMOST COMPLETE CURES

Are autistic children condemned to stay autistic for their whole life? Will they need lifelong care, even if certain treatments can substantially improve their state? Will they ever be able to have a normal life like their healthy peers? Is there a way to restore their normal brain function? In this chapter I will show that these children can be healed 100% and have a normal life again without requiring special services. Step by step I will go through their cases to show clearly how such a healing process will bring them to complete healing. When I ask the parents what percent their child is healed at a certain point of the treatment and they answer 70%, we have to realize that this is just a subjective evaluation. But if they say that the healing is complete and that their daughter or son is a normal child again at every level as any other child, that he or she can attend a regular school, does not have any problem interacting with other children, that there are no tics or obsessions anymore, that his or her emotional and mental life is balanced, that speech is normal again and all skills are age-appropriate, then we may assume that this child has completely healed from his disease.

The following case shows us that when all causations are resolved step by step and additional constitutional homeopathic remedies are used, 100% healing can be achieved.

Treatments with drugs are in essence material, which means that they are concentrations of certain substances like Ritalin, Concerta and Haloperidol. But unnatural drugs are unable to heal because they don't address the cause of the disease. At best, they just suppress the symptoms which are the outcome of the disease but not the disease itself. At the same time these drugs, because they are foreign to the body, cause multiple side-effects.

Natural substances are much more effective because they replace shortages of vitamins, minerals, fatty acids, proteins and enzymes to make the body function optimally. In our modern society, with its mostly denatured food supply, this has become an important issue. Supplements can often be used just to supply what is lacking, plus in higher doses they have a therapeutic effect. For example, very high doses of vitamin C can be used in the healing process of cancer. But these supplements can never replace healthy basic food. In this quantitative approach, significant improvements can also be attained by a gluten and casein free diet, a diet without sugar and milk, etc.

Therapies based on the behavioral approach, like the Sonrise and ABA therapy, also have their successes. These therapists have to struggle to work with a malfunctioning brain. Homeopathy is so effective, especially Isotherapy, because by its deep healing properties the brain can be brought back to its normal functioning. If these therapists could add homeopathic treatment simultaneously, they would probably find their work more effective.

With the endless possibilities that homeopathy offers us, with remedies made out of thousands of substances, we can heal that part that is inaccessible for the medical and supplement approaches. As earlier stated, autism is an accumulation of different causations that have made their imprints on the energetic level. Here homeopathy shows its full capacity to heal. The combination of Isotherapy (using the substance that caused the imprints in the vital energy of the patient) eventually followed by classical homeopathy or Inspiring Homeopathy, can heal an autistic child 100%. It is my dream that within one or two years all parents with an autistic child worldwide will know that their child can be healed or strongly improved with the method I describe in this book. This method shows also in an unmistakable way the causes of autism and of so many other behavioral problems in our young children.

Let us see step by step in the following cases exactly how this works.

Case of a combination of detoxification, classical homeopathy and orthomolecular support, three years treatment

Justin was 7 years old and diagnosed as PDD-NOS when I saw him for the first time in the summer of 2005. The dramatic change in his behavior took place when his parents took him to Kenya. He was then two and a half years old. He suddenly began having tantrums, turning his eyes away. This also happened during the night as if he were in another world. He never was an easy child, he was always crying as a baby and he would run in circles on the playground. But when the tantrums started, the parents knew that this was not normal. Such a change in behavior must have a reason, and I immediately suspected the tropical vaccinations he got just before the tantrums started (hepatitis A and yellow fever), plus Lariam, an oral anti malaria drug. He stayed in Kenya from April to December 2000.

Back home he got middle ear and throat infections with the usual rounds of antibiotics. This was May 2001, and one month later he had his tonsils and adenoids removed. But he had trouble coming out of the anesthesia. For a whole day he seemed to be in a trance and was unresponsive. Then at age four he got the usual DTPol and Neisvac-C shots. He then became very constipated for months. His stool had to be removed with enemas.

In 2004 he got another Hepatitis A shot. By that time he lived completely in his own world, with a lot of tantrums, and attended a special school for autistic children. He hardly was able to concentrate, spoke with one or two words, and was unable to tell a story. He saw only details, without being able to grasp a whole situation.

But this is only half of the story. As said before, he cried very often the first year and never slept during the day. He was bottle fed. He was full of tension, making fists with his hands. He suffered also from eczema from three months on (which was gone by the time of the consult).

It was not difficult to discover where all this came from. His mother had surgery in her third month of pregnancy for a benign lymph node in her neck, a long operation under general anesthesia and with antibiotics given preventively. This explains why he had so many problems when he got anesthesia himself at age two and a half. As a baby he already had diarrhea, which is still there, 4-5 times a day, sometimes solid, sometimes liquid. He also perspires profusely during the night, literally he is swimming in his perspiration as the parents express it. He has also a kind of herpes around his mouth and nose. All this indicates that his system is still reactive and that his body is trying to clear out toxins through his bowels and skin. His system is on survival mode so to say. His IQ is evaluated at 75, but for me this has no special value, because a blocked brain cannot function correctly. A virtuoso piano player cannot play Mozart with a broken finger; it has to heal first.

Treating more and more autistic children, I became aware also that the parents' history before the pregnancy should not be overlooked either. His mother had many courses of antibiotics for bronchial infections as a child and developed migraines from the age of 19 when she started birth control (which she used until she became pregnant). She also got a D&C with general anesthesia for a miscarriage shortly before her pregnancy with Justin. So there were many possible causations to detoxify.

On the mental and emotional level Justin had many typical autistic characteristics. He had poor social skills, as if he did not need others and did not understand other childrens' games. Nevertheless he liked to cuddle with his parents. He had no flexibility and was very obstinate. He was obsessed with numbers. He was reckless in the face of danger and was afraid of nothing. He loved to play with a Game Boy. Instructions addressed to a group passed him by completely. He ate everything but did not have a favorite food.

With all this information it was possible to make a good analysis of Justin's life story and to plan his step by step healing, i.e. the solution to all the causative factors that led to his autism. It can easily be understood that it will be a process not of months but of years to eliminate all the disturbances in his energetic system.

I retained the following causative elements: antibiotics used by his mother during childhood and her pregnancy with him, and by Justin himself during the first years of his life; then his mother's anesthesia during the pregnancy and that of her son at almost three years. With that we have to pay attention to his vaccinations, first to the yellow fever and hepatitis A shots after which his behavior changed completely, but also to the other usual vaccinations (Neisvac-C, MMR and DTPP/Hib) which he got in the first and second year of his life. Finally we keep in mind Lariam, a drug he took during six months in Kenya. Because autism is not provoked just by one factor but by an accumulation of different causations, the detoxification of all the factors should heal this boy completely. Experience taught that the detoxification of the cause which provoked the switch from a normal to an autistic child is not enough and will only give a partial improvement. The order in which this detoxification is done is not fixed and can be executed in a variable order. Mostly a reverse order is used, with the most recent cause healed first, but also the most probable and striking causations can be detoxified first. Later on, less probable factors can also be resolved to complete the healing process if necessary.

I started Justin's treatment with a course of Antibiotics (a homeopathic mixture of the most common antibiotics), every potency twice in 4 weeks and after a 2 weeks rest Nux vomica in 4 weeks to detoxify the anesthesia. Nux vomica is a wonderful homeopathic remedy for this, but is nevertheless not a perfect match. It is rather complicated to find out the specific anesthesia used and then to get the homeopathic remedy made from it. Fortunately there is also a mixture available with all kinds of anesthetics called General Anesthetics. At that time I was prescribing Nux vomica because I was not yet very familiar with its use, otherwise I certainly would have used it. Through experience this method of treatment for autism has step by step been improved. That is why I am able to present the CEASE method to the world, having learned from experience and always looking for a more successful approach.

Along with this he also was given the usual fat-soluble vitamin C (ascorbyl palmitate) and water soluble vitamin C with magnesium and zinc and fish oil. This orthomolecular treatment helps to make the healing process smoother and quicker.

On both courses he had severe fever blisters on his face, around his mouth, nose and eyes, indicating that the detoxification had started. He fell asleep more easily, and curiously enough he started to tell his dreams every morning. He also had pain in his abdomen on a regular basis. Before continuing to detoxify the yellow fever (Stamaril) I decide to start with Saccharum officinale 30C, twice a week, and Saccharum officinale D6, one tablet per day for two months, because of his bowel problems, the enormous sweating and his mental-emotional picture. During this treatment his speech was progressing, but he still had the fever blisters on his face, and his eczema came back over his whole body. His stool became more solid, but the sweating was not better. All eruptions during such a healing process have to be seen as temporary means that the body needs to detoxify and find a better balance. This means also that the disease is healing from more to less important organs, from the inside out. Suppressing these eruptions from outside with ointments just sabotages the body's efforts to heal and pushes it back to a deeper level again.

Then the Stamaril was given over 4 weeks. The parents talked about a breakthrough. The eczema, blisters and night sweats were much less, and he stopped biting his nails. But the real breakthrough took place on the mental and emotional level. He was more open, his empathy strongly increased, he was much more connected with his feelings and was upset if other people were suffering. He would react when his parents spoke to him. Saccharum off 30C also seemed to work better. His mood changed from rebellious to kind, he could easily be corrected, and he became more flexible. Finally he had no further abdominal pain and his stool was solid after many years of diarrhea. His concentration was still very bad, and he still had his strong obsession with numbers. At school he was teachable and his aggression was gone. His flexibility greatly increased. At this point the parents evaluated his healing at 60 or 70%, which is already an enormous improvement.

Then the Stamaril course was repeated and Saccharum was increased to a 200C once a week. During the Stamaril course his fever blisters increased again as during the first course. On the Saccharum officinale 200C he reacted quite violently: he became very rebellious and obsessive and the night perspiration increased again. The reason for such a strong aggravation was a misunderstanding; the parents gave the Saccharum twice a week instead of once a week. When this medication was stopped the aggravation disappeared quickly. On the second course of Stamaril, every potency was given until no reaction.

After that a big change took place in his energy. He became very insecure and had hardly any interest in the world around him; his empathy had gone again and he stopped showing his emotions. He was focusing on negativity. His speech had in contrary progressed and his interaction with other children was better. Is there reason to believe that he cannot be healed and that he will stay autistic for his whole life? Surely not; such waves in the healing process are not abnormal and a consequence of changing energies. Here homeopathy is again a master therapy to adapt to the new situation and to help him with the next step in the healing process. Not every step can be successful either, but all the important causations must be addressed.

I then put Justin on Carcinosinum cum Cuprum 30C, a homeopathic remedy that fits perfectly with his lack of self-confidence and obsessive behavior with lack of flexibility. The Saccharum officinale D6 once a day was continued to support his digestive system. When I saw the parents 4 months later there was some progress, especially his speech continued to develop, but his uncertainty had not really progressed. The parents had stopped the Carcinosinum cum Cuprum on their own after one month because they did not see much progress. These things happen and the homeopath just has to cope. At every consultation the reasons for good or bad results have to be evaluated carefully in order to lead the patient to complete healing.

So I put Justin again on the Carcinosinum cum Cuprum 30C, and because some of the Saccharum symptoms like the night sweating had increased again, I prescribed this remedy in an LM6 every day, except for the one day per week that he got his Carcinosinum cum Cuprum.

Three months later there was nice improvement. In the beginning of this treatment he became very emotional with a lot of crying. The parents were amazed at what he could do. He was more connected with the world around him and could make snappy observations. He started to experiment with all kind of things typical for his age. He was able to follow programs on TV, and his empathy came back again. He showed more emotions, sometimes being very sad. He even started to say 'she' when talking about his sister. His fever blisters almost disappeared. He still needed a lot of support, but he had more self confidence. Now I switched him to the 200C once a week of Carcinosinum cum Cuprum and to the LM12 of Saccharum officinale. I realized that we had not yet completed the detoxification of his vaccines, but as long as he was progressing with the actual medication it was wise to continue. Nevertheless there is a big chance that this process will get stuck somewhere because of a blockage caused by the vaccines or other causations that are still not resolved.

And indeed when I saw Justin and his parents four months later, the healing process had slowed down. Sure, he was able to express himself correctly and to tell a story that made sense, he was flexible and able to make a plan for himself for the day. Nevertheless he was still sweating a lot at night, and his obsession with numbers had not disappeared yet. The sweating showed that his system was still overloaded with toxins (the body was using the sweat as a way of eliminating them).

Then the detoxification continued with the Hepatitis A vaccine (Havrix), then the Neisvac-C, followed by the MMR and finally the DTPP/Hib, with a two week interval between every course of four weeks.

During the Hepatitis A course he became very obstinate and restless, but after the course these symptoms disappeared again spontaneously.

On the Neisvac-C course he had no reactions, but on the MMR there was clear progress in his cognitive skills. He started to ask questions and had more different interests. His obsessions become less for the first time and he was able to draw other pictures instead of series of numbers.

On the DTPP/Hib detoxification he became unbearable, was in a constant hurry, and wanted to try out everything that came up in his mind. Also the fever blisters on his face came back again. But after this detoxification he became very calm and flexible.

Then there was an intermezzo with a red and swollen finger around the nail. The family doctor prescribed antibiotics that again would set his healing process back. Fortunately homeopathy has good remedies for such infections. I prescribed for him Silicea D12 in water, a sip every hour for a week, and asked his parents to call with a report after 24 hours. The infection was then already better and after a week it was completely healed.

His school report was very positive: less angry; more able to have a conversation; understood more, listened better, got less frustrated, was able to follow instructions to the whole group. He was still behind with his vocabulary and with reading.

The conclusion of the parents after these four detoxifications was that there was a huge improvement. When I asked them how far the healing process had progressed, the father hesitated. He says: 'I would say 100%, but there is something that is still not as it should be to declare him 100% healed. He has little interest in the world around him. He has no hobbies, no ambition, he is not interested for example in learning to tie his shoes. He never asks why. He does not feel any need to nourish himself on the intellectual level.' His mother said: 'During the detoxification we had the impression that there was a breakthrough, but at the end he fell back as if there is still something missing.'

Then I realized that he was now in a state as if he were still half under anesthesia and I remembered that the detoxification of the anesthesia with Nux vomica did not give the expected improvement. Therefore I decided to start right away with Opium, another remedy used in homeopathy to detoxify anesthesia. Opium has the same dullness and lack of interest. I kept in mind that the MMR and DTTP/Hib should be still repeated at least one more time and that the detoxification of Lariam should also be done to complete the whole treatment.

The course of Opium over 4 weeks had indeed the expected and desired results. First he became rebellious again, but soon he became more alert and started to play football with other children even if he didn't know them. His father went with him to an amusement park and really had the feeling of having a normal child who enjoyed all the attractions and was able to stand in line and wait his turn nicely. It was as if the haze had finally been lifted from his brain. Even his teacher was surprised that he could read calmly and retain everything he had read.

Now we approached the final goal of his healing process, that is the complete healing with the restoration of all the damage that was unconsciously done to a healthy boy. These last steps I will guide him through also and make sure that nothing has been overlooked that can still harm him in his functioning on the mental, emotional and physical level.

When the MMR course was repeated, his parents said it was like a wonder. After three years his profuse sweating at night stopped suddenly. He also took more initiative.

Then the DTPP course provoked a strong reaction. He became quite obsessive again and his behavior was more autistic-like, as if he got his wires crossed and got stuck in his established patterns. After the course he improved again, but that meant that both the MMR and especially the DTPP had to be repeated. Apparently the information in his energy which is built up with the MMR and DTPP energy is still there, otherwise there would not have been such a strong reaction. Nevertheless both courses improved his concentration and at school he was really doing his very best. Only his verbal capacities like understanding and speaking in complete sentences were still weak.

The course with MMR did not give further reaction, but on the DTPP he reacted again, especially on the 1M and 10M. His blisters disappeared completely. He became talkative and started to write down stories, showing his creativity. His speech is nevertheless still far behind compared to his classmates. Now he is open and alert and his empathy has increased a lot. He has become independent also, riding his bike alone or taking the bus alone. He suddenly started to tie his shoes also. He enjoys going on holiday. The only detoxification left on our list is Lariam. But the parents reconfirm without any hesitation that they don't have an autistic child any more, just a child with some speech and language problems. Will the detoxification of Lariam give a boost to that also? Time will give us the answer.

When I reread his healing story, I realize that nowadays based on many experiences with these treatments I work more systematically, preferring mostly to finish all the detoxifications first and then pass to general homeopathy to complete the process if necessary. Sometimes for the comfort of the parents, the child or the school, a well chosen homeopathic remedy can be given in between or along with the detoxification courses. Also detoxification of a substance has to be repeated as long as there are reactions. Reactions means that the information is still in the energetic system and should be cleared out completely before passing to the next. When this is not done properly this can still be repaired later as I have done in this case.

Testimonial of Justin's parents - From calculator to story writer

Our son Justin is almost 11 years old now; he has been diagnosed as PDD-NOS and attends a special school for autistic children. Our son has already been treated for more than three years by Dr. Smits. Our initial request was to improve especially his concentration and language. Justin had problems with reading and speech in general, had difficulties to evaluate a situation (action and reaction), had difficulties to play with other children. Sometimes it was difficult to make contact with him and he could panic and become angry when he could not take stock of the situation. He would easily grumble or have tantrums. He always was in a hurry when he had to perform tasks at school. He was completely obsessed by numbers, so severely that it blocked somehow his normal development. He could fill notebooks with numbers for hours. With that he had several physical complaints like eczema, liquid stools, night sweats, and many blisters in his face around mouth and nose.

Nowadays Justin has no tantrums and can make contact without any problem. He can easily evaluate a situation and does not have problems changing from one situation to another; you don't have to prepare him beforehand. His constant hurry has disappeared when performing tasks at school. He is less distracted and he is not sitting any more in a box, but at a table next to another child. He has become more social … he stopped filling up notebooks with numbers but is writing stories he invents himself.

Recently we evaluated his healing at 100% concerning his autistic behavior. What is still left is a language problem. It is as if through the treatment of Dr. Smits his autism has completely disappeared. As Dr. Smits says: it is like an onion and we take off a layer until we reach the core. Now we will focus on his language problem and that is why he will go after the summer holidays to a special secondary school for children with language and speech problems without disturbances in behavior.

As parents we are very happy with this situation. Justin is a sweet and happy boy, loved by everybody. He sleeps well, eats well, does not use any medication except the homeopathic ones, practices sport and feels well. We can take him everywhere and have a normal family life. From his physical complaints almost nothing is left. What is still left is only linked with his speech and language problems and not with any autistic feature.

Thank you Dr. Smits for all we have achieved so far.

Case of Tom, rapid healing

The complete healing process of an autistic child generally takes 2 to 4 years depending on how complicated the case is, how many causations have to be treated, and how fast the remedies work. The case of Tom, age 6, has taken only one year. He was diagnosed with ASS (Autistic Spectrum Syndrome) half a year before. There is no breaking point in his life story. He had no special reactions to his vaccinations. The only thing to notice is that he had three Hepatitis B shots from the age of eight months, which is not usual in Holland, but is standard in Belgium where they live.

His mother received progesterone to become pregnant, her pregnancy and delivery were uneventful, and she breastfed him for four months. The first year Tom hardly ever had a cold, but then he had colds very frequently until three and a half years, which indicates that his system was overloaded and needed to detoxify. From the age of two he started to cough, which was successfully treated with chiropractic.

In his case it all happened gradually. He was a dreamer and turned the wheels of his cars and did not learn routine gestures. At school when he was three years old the teacher kept asking his mother if he could hear well, as he did not follow instructions properly. His fine motor skills got more and more behind, although his gross motor skills were within the normal range. He never asked for something to eat or to drink and he never asked why. His food desires were simple; he would like to eat only lasagna at dinner. Until age four he refused to eat hard food and he loved sweets. His speech developed normally. His parents both got tropical vaccinations eight years before he was born: DTP, Typhoid and Hepatitis A.

In the case of Tom there are no indications for any specific causation. So I started the treatment with the detoxification of his vaccines with short courses of 15 days followed by one week break between the different vaccines during which he received one dose of Saccharum off.

30C, plus three times per day Vitamin C with magnesium and zinc, ascorbyl palmitate and fish oil. After two courses of MMR, Neisvac-C, hepatitis B and DTPP/Hib without clear reactions there was some progress but not very striking. The main thing was that he was doing well at school and that he could go to the next grade. The overall improvement so far was estimated at 30%; his comprehension seemed better. Then I decided to treat him with Choriongonadotrophine, the hormone the mother took to become pregnant, along with Saccharum off. 200C once a week. First the DTPP/Hib was given for the second time because that one was not yet given for the second time at the second consultation. During the DTPP/Hib course he was easily tired and a little bit irritated, reactions he had also on the other courses.

On a 4 week course of the Choriongonadotrophine he had no reactions, but after these detoxifications there was a spectacular recovery. As so often happens, we don't know which remedy was responsible or whether it was in the combination. He changed from a zombie to a teachable, active and receptive little boy. He was able to follow regular schooling, his fine motor skills became much better, he understood everything, was alert and enjoyed life. It was as if his mind is open again, the parents say. The interaction with other children was normal again, his sleep became quiet, and he had no more anxieties at night. He also became potty trained during the night. The parents declared him 100% cured. I kept him on Saccharum off. 1M, once every two weeks for the next half year.

Case of Siem, careful detoxification of all causative factors leading to complete healing

The story of Siem is very special and it is worthwhile to tell his story. He is the boy with autism on the DVD about vaccination damage *(described end of the book)*. He was 9 years old when I saw him in February 2005. Almost four years have passed, and during that time he changed from a severely autistic child to a completely healed wonderful adolescent who is in many aspects wiser than his peers. When his parents were interviewed for the DVD, he also asked to tell his story for the camera. He then said the famous words which have so impressed me: *'It is as if I am in a second life.'*

First I want to express my sincere admiration for his mother, who fought like a tiger to help her son recover from this horrible disease which is still labeled incurable. Certainly she was criticized by psychologists, school officials, and other parents. She was told to seek psychological help to learn to accept her son's diagnosis. But throughout her son's whole healing process, she never lost her unshakable belief that her son would one day become a normal child able to develop all the wonderful talents he was born with. And that day has come, I will tell you his story. His mother reminds me of another mother who has also fought for her son and has written a very inspiring book of their story: Jenny McCarthy in *Louder Than Words*, which is a bestseller in the USA. Her book must have encouraged many other mothers to do the same and fight for their child. Like Siem's mother, she had to face enormous challenges alone, because the father and husband was not able to handle the whole situation and left.

Siem was a completely normal child until age four. He was healthy, cuddling and calm and interacted well with other children. He walked at 13 months and bicycled at two and a half years (the latter is normal for Holland although not for the US). His speech was at a good level. He was a joy for his parents.

At age four, one week after the DTPol shot, he suddenly regressed and did not know anymore how to put his jacket on the coat rack, how to dress or undress. Even the simplest act became problematic. He became extremely anxious, not wanting to go to the toilet alone. Soon he became constipated, a common symptom in autistic children. He wanted only yoghurt and crackers to eat, refused warm food, soft food and meat. He immediately started to give up when his mother insisted. Siem had become a shadow of himself, Siem was not Siem anymore. Half a year later he was diagnosed with autism.

How could a completely healthy child suddenly lose his abilities at age four and become severely autistic? Which deep disturbance was responsible for this complete transformation on the physical, mental and emotional level? Most children become autistic around one and a half or two years old. Siem's case is quite exceptional and can give us valid information about what caused the blockage of his brain with the loss of his personality and physical abilities. Because everything started one week after the DTPol shot, this immunization surely plays an important role in his setback. Nevertheless through experience I have learned that the detoxification of the DTPol alone will not bring Siem back completely. His case will show clearly that this shot could only be destructive because there were already several other causes that had damaged his energy without producing any development disorder. In fact the DTPol was like the last block that makes the whole tower fall down. This theory has been confirmed by the case of Siem and many other cases. To heal him 100%, several detoxifications have to be executed carefully. His case also shows how important it is to have a thorough and complete case history with all the facts. If you miss one factor, the final healing can be missed also.

His parents refused the repetition of the DTPol and MMR shots that he normally would have had at age nine. They also did not allow him to be vaccinated against meningoccus-C, which was introduced in Holland at that time. For his mother, there was no doubt that the DTPol shot was responsible for her son's autism, regardless of what the authorities and doctors said. In any case she felt the official care was worthless. She is still offended that a special education teacher stated that she was in severe denial and that she should accept her son's fate. She realized that she could not expect much from the official assistance and had already decided at an early stage to take charge of her own child's treatment.

After spending a whole day in her son's class, she was exhausted by the horrible noise and hyperactivity of the autistic and ADHD children. Now she understood why Siem lay on the floor after school and just wanted to rest. Siem was hypersensitive to noise and crowds. His mother decided to keep him home and to teach him herself. She only got permission to keep him home for half a day. From that time on Siem only went to school in the morning, and in the afternoon his mother would teach him for about an hour. In ten months time he caught up on a year and a half of school.

In addition, his mother had already put him on a gluten and sugar free diet and gave him organic food, vitamin C, fish oil and a multi vitamin and mineral pill. These interventions alone improved him a lot. He suffered less from his phobias and was able to go out of the house again. He still had frequent pains in his abdomen and remained a picky eater, refusing any new food. He was still anxious, with many worries. Especially at night he had a strong fear of being alone and could not stay alone in a room for even a second. He was afraid of insects, any change, the unknown, and the dark. He had nightmares every night and would slip into his parents' bed. His grandmother passed away two years earlier; he would still see her and other light beings. Now he was also afraid to become old himself and to die. With that he had an enormous fear of failure and was an extreme perfectionist. When just one little line was wrong in his drawing, he would rip up the paper and start the drawing over. His concentration was fleeting.

The logical treatment at that point was to detoxify first the DTPol shot which he got at age four and which was the turning point in his life. I decided to take at least 8 weeks, giving every potency four times. This first treatment caused tremendous reactions of fever and diarrhea on every new potency, but by the time each potency was given four times, the reactions had already faded away. He still had abdominal pains and felt nauseous.

Since that course he had super days with high alertness, normal participation in all activities at home, and was more sympathetic. He was again able to go to the bathroom alone. His fear of failure considerably improved, and he became curious. At this point his mother evaluated the progress at 50-60%, although his father was more pessimistic or maybe realistic and gave it a 30-40%.

I decided then to continue with the detoxification of the MMR and DTPol/Hib, because most likely the early disturbances had already taken place with the first vaccinations. Along with the detoxification he received Saccharum off. D6 to support his digestive system. His reaction on the MMR was quite strong with restlessness, lack of concentration and extreme anxiety. After this MMR he quickly improved again, his anxieties decreased again, his concentration was better, and he had fewer fits of crying. He began playing in the street and brought a new friend home for the first time. He was able to handle changes in his daily routine. His awareness increased; he asked for the first time, after three years, why he had to take swimming lessons with special needs children and why he had to go to a special school. When he got his DTPol/Hib course, he relapsed again, was very nauseous and vomited easily.

Then his mother told me that his first vaccination was a DTPP/Hib, that he got whooping cough after that shot, and that he got finally only DTPol/Hib shots. So I decided at that point to detoxify his DTPP/Hib shot to clear out that disturbance too, but he did not react on that course. Then the MMR course was repeated three times over 3 months time, with gradual general improvement, but his digestive problems continued to give trouble with nausea and miserable appetite. Saccharum off. 200C was not able to change that either. When I asked his mother what 8 months of homeopathy have brought, she said: 'It is phenomenal.' Nevertheless important progress still had to be made. He was still very uncertain, was unable to work independently, and still had eating problems. He would get too stressed out at school, then he would relax during the holidays and feel much better.

Then he was treated with Carcinosinum cum Cuprum and Vernix caseosa over a period of two years to boost his self-confidence and to make him less sensitive to external stimuli. With this treatment he gradually improved; his digestive problems disappeared, except his abdominal pains after meals. However he remained a fragile and anxious boy who felt unhappy at school. He also had regular nightmares.

I continued to look for information to understand why he was so fragile and why he has still not completely recovered. During this time I gradually realized through other cases how important the period before pregnancy can be also. Then I learned that his mother had a general breakdown two years before her pregnancy with Siem. It all started with an infection in the root of a tooth. She had two or three rounds of antibiotics but still needed more. She had already had many rounds of antibiotics in her life for sinusitis. She was so weak that she could not hold a knife, was unable to read a newspaper, lost her way when travelling on the train, and spent about a year and a half in bed. She also had many food allergies. She also had swollen glands, in other words typical symptoms of mononucleosis, although there was no definitive diagnosis.

No doubt she passed these energetic disturbances to her son at least partially, and that we have to detoxify these imbalances to heal Siem completely. We started the treatment with the homeopathic remedy Mononucleosis in a four week course. Unexpectedly his reactions were not very clear, but during the whole course he was tired, not alert and slept deeply as if unconscious. His nose ran profusely, indicating that the detoxification had started. So the course was repeated a second time. On the 1M potency he was extremely tired and felt ill. He had to stay home for two weeks, mostly in bed or on the couch.

After that there was a spectacular reversal. At school there was a miracle, his mother said. Suddenly he was able to do everything without any problem. His concentration, his understanding in calculation and his logical thinking improved greatly. He became much more independent. His anxieties — which did not leave him for so many years and made life so difficult for him and his family — were almost completely gone. At home there were the same changes and he was no longer a picky eater. His energy increased enormously. It was hard to believe that he could make such a leap forward just by eliminating the mononucleosis energy. It was clear that the main cause of his autism had to be found in this disease. I realized that his healing process would have been much quicker if this information had been available from the beginning. But I also realize that every case I have seen in the last three years has contributed to a better understanding of this disease and its successful treatment.

While detoxifying the antibiotics he felt ill again with flu and his nose was running again. To be sure that everything was eradicated a second course of the remedy Antibiotics was given, but there were no clear reactions anymore. Then a third course of the remedy Mononucleosis was given with no reactions. With that we can conclude that this part of his healing has been successfully completed.

Then at a school camp he was bitten by a dog, not very severely but the director wanted him to be vaccinated again against tetanus. Siem protested violently but he could not convince his teachers, and the doctor was already called. Completely panicked he escaped and hid for hours in the attic. Meanwhile his mother had been phoned and immediately forbade the tetanus shot. At home everybody was proud of him.

When I saw him some months later he had become more stable, the fragile expression had completely disappeared. The school was too easy for him now, he performed too high with scores of 90 to 100%.

He had also become the teacher's aide in his class, a task he performed with much enthusiasm and skillfulness. His mother did not want him to change school in the middle of the year, but it was clear that he had completely outgrown this type of school. Next year he will start at a normal secondary school, he is ready for that.

His complete healing has taken three and a half years, although it could have been completed in only about two years with the right approach and right information. But even if it took extra time the results are wonderful and can help other autistic children to heal also. In this way the CEASE therapy developed to an effective tool to stop the scourge of this disease for the children and for the parents.

Testimonial of Siem's mother

Siem is the youngest of three children and is thriving well. He is a jolly toddler, likes to play outside home with his friends and is fond of animals. Once at the primary school (4 years) he makes contact easily because he is quick to laugh and is easy going.

A few months later Siem changes drastically. He becomes silent and absent-minded. He is scared to go out of home. He becomes fearful of the dark and insects. He is afraid to sleep and becomes intolerant of all kinds of foods with severe constipation. After a half year he can no longer perform simple tasks, he no longer knows how to put his coat on the coat hooks or what he should do in the bathroom. He now eats only crackers and yoghurt. He is constantly ill and has a stomach ulcer and bowel inflammation. His constipation has become a major problem, he usually has a spontaneous bowel movement only once every three weeks.

His jolly face has become pale and grave and his brilliant eyes look now like glass marbles. He looks through his eyes in the outer world, but there is no connection any more. This always present little boy is sitting now as a puppet on my lap with his head on my neck and I carry him all day around, because walking has become too exhausting for him.

After half a year we get his final diagnosis: classic autism and probably retarded. With that we get the advice to find a good place for him because of his restricted development expectations.

After a couple of years at a special school with problem oriented counseling Siem is not progressing. He is unable to perform a simple task independently and his constipation has become a nightmare. He suffers from phobic anxieties. He is unable to function in his class, also because of the unpredictable behavior of other children who have all more or less severe behavior problems.

Then we decide to keep him home and to set to work ourselves. We organize a special learning and development program. To prepare him for this we start with a wheat, milk and sugar free diet. With that he gets some herbs from his usual therapist to heal the acute bowel inflammation and to improve his constitution. His alertness then increases and he begins to perform simple tasks. We teach him to write and read, to tell time and the days of the week. He has difficulties with calculation. Nevertheless his bad concentration and severe constipation stay a major problem.

Because of his autism many activities are only possible with careful planning. For example he is able to start swimming lessons and to learn the basic principles with much patience and intense coaching. He only makes contact with his brother and sister and cannot live for even moment without me, his mother. I understand and translate his demands and try to realize them for him.

Then I find the site of Dr. Tinus Smits and contact him. Finally a doctor who is supporting my suspicion that the relapse in Siem's development is caused by vaccination. We start with the detoxification of his vaccines and the administration of vitamin C and fish oil. During the detoxification of the MMR Siem falls sick, high fever and violent diarrhea. Giving the higher potencies it even becomes worse, but after the course my child has profoundly changed. He takes his coat from the coat hooks and goes playing in the street. If I want to go with him, he says with a laugh that he is old enough to go alone. Amazing!

His learning is progressing constantly. He still has violent reactions on the detoxification of the antibiotics and mononucleosis, which I have got two years before his birth. His autistiform behavior disappears. He reacts with flexibility to changes. He becomes a social and balanced teen who meanwhile takes the bus to a regular school by himself. In the first class of the secondary school (13 years) he has been chosen as class representative, his grades have so far been 80% and higher. He is swimming like an otter (Dutch expression!) and is mountain biking every week. The teacher at school has discovered his musical talents and Siem is now taking drum lessons. His teacher is excited about the speed he is learning new things and his progressions. He plays comfortably in front of people at an open day at school.

Every day I am amazed about the catching up of his retardation that nobody believed that ever could be possible.

Siem himself says: 'It is as if I am in a second life. It is completely different from before.'

Monique, mother of Siem

Case of Stijn, rapid healing by detoxification

In the following case we see a clear setback after a double vaccination (MMR and Neisvac-C) at 14 months of age during a common cold. The detoxification of all his vaccines led finally to complete healing. These results were obtained in only 8 months which is an exceptionally short period. The parents are amazed.

Stijn was a seven year old boy who had been diagnosed autistic (ASD) with developmental delays last year. But he knew everything about trains in the greatest detail and he knew all the cathedrals of Europe by heart, not really common for normal intelligent children let alone special needs children. This indicates that he had been an intelligent child whose brain was blocked, leaving some parts untouched or even in a hyperactive state. His social skills were quite good, but he had strong obsessions, lack of self-confidence and a strong rigidity.

Up to 14 months he did not have major health problems and was thriving quite well. His parents lived a rather healthy life, but were not very aware of the dangers of vaccinations. Pregnancy was uneventful, but at eight months the waters broke and delivery was provoked with oxytocin. He was not breastfed, and the bottle made him vomit and cry a lot. Nonetheless, he was a joyful and healthy child.

Everything changed after the MMR, according to the parents. However, my inspection of his vaccination record revealed that with the MMR he also got his Neisvac-C vaccination. For reasons that are unclear this last shot had been given a second time shortly after the first one. Moreover, these shots were given when he had a common cold, which constitutes a higher risk for post-vaccination health problems. After these vaccinations the expression in his eyes changed completely. He became glassy-eyed, as if the life suddenly had slipped away out of his body. He became self-absorbed and lost his usual *joie de vivre*. He retired into his own world, developed rigid play patterns, had no interest in new toys and had to always take the same route to school or he would start screaming. His speech had not been affected, and he was able to play with other children with humor and good interaction.

In this case vaccination seemed to be the major cause of his disability. The treatment was started with Neisvac-C over 4 weeks in 4 different potencies as usual. To lower the oxidative stress in his brain he was given ascorbyl palmitate 500mg 3 times per day 2 capsules and an ascorbate containing zinc and magnesium, 1000mg 3 times per day, plus fish oil 500mg twice per day.

The result of this detoxification was little short of a miracle. First he had a detox reaction during the treatment: protruded tongue, blank stare, and diarrhea. At the 10M he became angry again just as he had some years back shortly after the vaccinations. He flapped his hands, had a glassy-eyed look and was unreachable. But shortly after an enormous turnaround occurred and he once again became the little sunshine in the house. He was easily accessible again and understood everything. At school the big transformation had not gone unnoticed: he was able to follow instructions in an appropriate way. His mother evaluated the improvement at 70%.

These aggravations of the symptoms that first appeared shortly after the Neisvac-C show clearly that there was a connection between these symptoms and the shot itself. Sometimes these reactions are as strong as after the real shot with brain-cry, loss of brilliance in the eyes, fever, etc. Frequently parents report after the detoxification of the vaccines that the brilliance in the eyes has come back again. This is a meaningful sign, because the eyes are the doorway to the mind.

After two weeks the whole treatment was repeated in the same way. Again he had a clear reaction. On the 30C he was very tired and his concentration was very low. On the 1M his reaction was even more pronounced. One hour after the two tiny granules had been given, his eyes spread wide open, became red and teary as if inflamed and he started to blink with his left eye for the next two weeks. On the 10M he improved again and, as his mother said, a 'new child' was born. He played with more imagination and he adored horseplay and cuddling. He also had a new close friend.

Nevertheless, his concentration was bad, he had become more restless, had problems with falling asleep and woke up easily in the middle of the night. Every homeopath will easily recognize the picture of Saccharum officinale in these symptoms, but I preferred repeating the Neisvac-C course a third time to completely clean up its imprint as there were still strong reactions on the second course.

This time there were no detox reactions, but the progress was considerable. The good news was that he could stay at the school he was attending because he was now able to follow standard instructions. His obsessions completely disappeared and he no longer had a major interest in trains. He began shooting up in height and lost four teeth. Some problems remained. He still had poor body awareness and sometimes put his sweater on wrong. He was also unsteady on his feet. He still had difficulties falling asleep and his self-confidence was low. Rather than treat these problems with a specific homeopathic remedy, I preferred first treating the MMR and DTPP/Hib vaccinations.

On the MMR he did not have any specific reaction, he continued to function well. Then the DTPP/Hib course was started. On the 200C he had diarrhea with black fragments. When the whole course was repeated a second time again he had the same reaction on the 200C, which indicates that the main disturbance of this vaccine was located in this patient at the 200C level. Apart from these reactions he made a final leap to complete healing. His self-confidence grew considerably, and at school he became the best in the class in reading. He was even amazed at how he had behaved when he was still autistic, an incredible increase in his self-awareness. His parents are astonished about what happened with their son. 'We have our son back after seven years and there is no room for further improvement,' they said.

Case of Timo, diagnosed with classic autism, never vaccinated!
It would be a mistake to accuse only vaccines of causing autism, as I have stated earlier. Certainly vaccines are the main cause but not the only one, and other toxins can also accumulate to finally make a child autistic.

Timo was three and a half years old when I first saw him with his mother. His general development was far behind and had been evaluated at the ten month level. He could not talk, but grabbed his mother by her hand if he wanted something. He could not stand to wait even a second when he wanted something. He became angry if he was not satisfied immediately, with a tantrum that could last for 90 minutes; he would cry loudly, hit his parents and bang his head against them. Afterwards he would be very tired. Before he was one year old he had already started to bang his head in his bed and still did this to fall asleep. He was also aggressive toward himself. He would pinch his cheeks and scratch them open. It was almost impossible to correct him. If his mother became angry at him, he would be ill for three days and play victim. His hair never had been cut because he would panic completely.

Timo had hardly any eye-contact, but he noticed everything and constantly looked around. His motor skills were well developed. He is a hot child and loves to go without a shirt. He sweated profusely on his head and his neck during sleep. He easily got tired and wanted to lie down with his pacifier. He loved music, especially classical music. He would not play with his toys but would put them all in a certain order that was logical for him. He had hardly any fantasy life. At eight months his mother knew that something was different, and at 14 months she knew that he was autistic.

She had a good pregnancy, but frequently got the flu during which she used a Xylomethazolin nasal spray, plus she smoked six to eight cigarettes per day. Her son was born almost two weeks late, but the delivery was spontaneous and easy. His mother had postpartum depression after her first pregnancy a year and a half earlier. She had just as severe a depression this time and did not know how to handle her child. Six months after her first baby she was pregnant again when she was still in a miserable state. She nursed Timo for five or six weeks but had to stop because of cracked nipples. At ten weeks he had whooping cough which was healed in three days with a homeopathic remedy (Drosera). She never had him vaccinated because her eldest daughter got convulsions and muscular contractions after a vaccination. She had had a difficult childhood herself and left home to live with her grandmother because she was a difficult child. At seventeen she had a violent friend who abused her. She smoked marijuana and even a few times, she says, she took cocaine. Completely exhausted she returned to live with her parents.

Timo had already had some homeopathic treatment before I saw him, which improved his eye-contact and made him more open. I put him on ascorbyl palmitate, an ascorbate with zinc and magnesium and on fish oil. The first step in his treatment was to detoxify the Xylomethazolin in four weeks. Typically 36 hours after the administration of a Xylomethazolin potency he got abdominal pain with diarrhea. Already during this first course with many repetitions of the 1M and 10M, his understanding would increase a lot, and his mother would be able to get through to him more easily. His eye contact was much better and his speech became understandable because his articulation improved. On the other hand he had more problems with his stool; even a soft stool came out with difficulty. On the second course of Xylomethazolin he had no clear reactions, but Timo was nevertheless much clearer in his head, he understood everything, and was able to use more words, although he was still far behind in speech. He became a happy and radiant boy again. His reactions were quicker also. The eye contact was strongly improved. But he was still rigid and still had obsessive behavior.

Then I wanted to find out the role of tobacco smoking during the pregnancy. So the detoxification of tobacco was done with a course of Tabacum (the homeopathic remedy made from tobacco) over four weeks. The first course was a real drama, his mother said. Timo was very irritated and angry for hours and he was extremely aggressive: he hit, bumped his parents with his head to hurt them, and he shrieked all the time. But the parents did not doubt the usefulness of this therapy because they had already seen great improvements from the detoxification of Xylomethazolin and they were determined to get their child back again completely. On a second course of Tabacum, Timo only reacted on the 10M. After these two courses I saw Timo with his mother for a follow-up. He had made considerable progress on different levels and the overall improvement was evaluated at 60%. His eye contact was close to the normal level. His anger had improved enormously, and when he got angry he was able to snap out of it more easily. The head banging had almost ceased and he had stopped pinching his cheeks. His energy had also improved. He was able to complete tasks, and his speech had started to develop. He even referred to himself as 'me' in sentences, and he was able to indicate verbally what he liked and disliked. But he still ran away from his parents when not held by the hand.

I decide to repeat the Tabacum course a third time and to get the maximum benefit out of this treatment, to eradicate completely the damage that his mother's smoking had caused. During summer vacation his mother did not give the Tabacum course, because her son felt so well and she wanted to enjoy her child without risking more aggravations. When I saw Timo at the end of October she had just started again with the 30C. If there are no more reactions on this third course of Tabacum, he will be switched to a course of Cannabis (the homeopathic remedy made from marijuana) over 8 weeks, and the final touch will be cocaine in homeopathic doses.

With all this he will be probably healed completely, eventually with a finishing touch of Inspiring or Classical Homeopathy. What I wanted to show in the case of this unvaccinated autistic child is that we always have to look for the causation — and that these causations have to be there. No child will become autistic without special causations. Through the step by step resolution of causative factors it is possible to bring these children completely back again to good physical, emotional and mental health. This method is so certain in its outcome that it is no exaggeration to postulate here that this child will heal completely.

Complete healing with classical homeopathy
It is my experience, and therefore also my conviction, that classical homeopathy (giving a single remedy based on the totality of the patient's symptoms) is often not able to heal autism completely. If it could, homeopathy would already be famous for resolving the scourge of autism that is afflicting the world. Our results in classical homeopathy are too inconsistent. Classical homeopathy sometimes gives spectacular results (for example see *Impossible Cure* by Dr. Amy Lansky, the story of her son's cure of autism). Initially I was also trying to heal these children with classical homeopathy or rather with Inspiring Homeopathy. But after the administration of the 30C and 200C, the higher potencies did not work anymore, because further healing was blocked by the imprints of specific causative factors, which mostly could be cleared only with Isotherapy. Homeopathy can only work if the administered remedy resonates with the energy of the patient. That means that the information from both sides has to be the same. If a certain toxic substance has left an imprint in patient's energy, its isotherapeutic equivalent is the perfect remedy to provoke this vital resonance. That is why Isotherapy has finally proved to

be the preferential approach to heal autism. Nowadays I consider classical homeopathy and Inspiring Homeopathy much more as the polish at the end or in between the isotherapeutic treatment rather than the treatment itself. Nevertheless it cannot be denied that in rare cases complete healing can be achieved. Apparently in these cases a constitutional approach can restore the patient's energy to complete balance. Here follows such a case, in which I started right away with the classical approach and it was successful up to the end.

Case healed solely with classical homeopathy

Thomas was ten years old when at his first appointment in 2005. He had been diagnosed as autistic (ASD). Already when he was one year old his parents had the impression that something was not right. At kindergarten he did not participate in activities and there was no contact at all.

There were no significant events in his health history in infancy. He was breastfed for 10 months, after which he developed eczema in the bends of his arms and legs. At one year he developed sleeping problems with incessant crying and refusal to go to bed, which caused sleepless nights for his parents. Up until the age of eight, his parents would let him come into their bed to sleep. He was vaccinated according to the national vaccination program. After each shot he completely panicked.

Nowadays he still is difficult to reprimand, and punishment simply does not work. He has trouble when things are imposed and has difficulty expressing his thoughts. His speech and understanding are above average. His social skills with other children are well developed, but with adults he has problems. In difficult situations he scratches himself. Emotionally he is a very closed child. He always has warm hands and cold feet; he wants a hot water bottle in his bed. He has little self-confidence and often says, 'Oh, I can't do that.' He is frustrated that he cannot be the best or get a high mark. He has already stayed back twice in school. He has poor concentration and is unable to stick with a task. He can become angry from powerlessness. He is especially gifted in drawing. But he is very precise and many of his drawings end up in the wastebasket. Since he was weaned he became a picky eater, saying that he is not hungry. He is oversensitive to wheat. He is quite thirsty and loves sour foods like lemons, mustard, pickles, cocktail onions, and vinegar.

In the winter he becomes pale with repeated flus and with episodes of difficult breathing. His eczema also gets worse. He has cracks in the corner of his mouth.

I started his treatment with Carcinosinum 30C twice a week, to boost his self-confidence because low self-esteem is what he suffers from the most. With that he gets fish oil, ascorbate with zinc and magnesium, 3 times 2 grams per day and Saccharum officinale D6 one tablet per day to heal his digestive system and to avoid food restrictions. In the margin I wrote 'vaccination and food' to remind myself to come back to these factors if the classical remedy gives poor results.

Two and a half months later he was much better already, and everybody around him noticed it. He felt all right, his eczema and cracks completely disappeared, and the skin of his back was no longer like sandpaper. His paleness has been replaced by a healthy color and he had no more headaches. There had taken place a marvelous turnaround, and his mother said she was astonished. Thomas felt much more confident, was even able to study for a test independently without panicking, had better concentration, went out with his parents for the first time, and had hardly any more outbursts of anger. He also was more accepted by his peers.

The Carcinosinum 30C was still continued for one month and then replaced by the 200C once a week. An episode of cough and mucus in

135

his chest was easily tackled with a water solution of the Carcinosinum 200C, one sip every hour for three days.

Three months later he had again progressed nicely. At school he was performing much better and had no further difficulties at his grade level. His main problem was now communication. He was unable to participate in a football game, he stayed alone on the field, isolating himself rather than joining a team. He simply did not understand what was expected from him. He had problems interacting with strangers. He also stopped going out with his parents. I decided to put him then on Carcinosinum 1M, once every two weeks, and to add Saccharum off. 30C three times in 2 weeks, because Saccharum acts so nicely on the social and emotional qualities. Here probably the pure classical homeopaths would go up the wall, continuing the treatment with the same remedy or looking for another remedy, with the risk of jeopardizing complete healing with too many remedies. I put again in the margin: 'Vaccinations!'

Four months later he had become quiet and had finished his best school year ever, in spite of the bad results that were predicted. His social skills had not yet improved substantially, but because of the overall improvement I decided to continue both remedies, Carcinosinum in a 1M and Saccharum off. in a 200C, both in alternation over two weeks. He made steady progress. Carcinosinum was upgraded to a 10M and Saccharum off. to a 1M, again in alternation over two weeks.

When I saw Thomas for a follow-up four months later, his parents declared him completely healed. 'It is unbelievable,' they say, 'that he tells us what happened at school and he can express his feelings nicely. When we sit on the couch together and Thomas is in bed, we look at each other and say: "Is this our child?"' Formerly he was like a doll, now he is a lively boy of his age with good results at school and a lot of activities outside of school. He has a lively social life with lots of friends. His memory has also clearly improved. He has become independent and takes responsibility for himself. He is able to argue and to reason with logic like children of his age, surprising his parents. He can accept a refusal from his parents without becoming angry. Unfortunately he has not become a good football player and his father seems to have accepted this now. In the meantime, the cracks in the corners of his mouth and a spot of eczema in his left elbow have come back. This happens more often under stress, his parents say. Is this still a residue of vaccinations? It is impossible to know at this point of his treatment. If physically he is bothered later on by these skin problems I will surely consider detoxifying his vaccinations. Finally I put him on Carcinosinum and Saccharum off. both in a 10M for the next six months to avoid regression and heal him at a very deep level. These results were achieved in less than two years.

Testimonial of Thomas' parents

Our son Thomas was born January 1995. The period of being a baby went by normally, however after his first year he started to be difficult during night time (crying a lot and not wanting to sleep). Those sleeping-problems stayed for many years on end. Also as a toddler he had abnormal behavior. At the nursery he made no contact with other children and those in charge could not handle him.

An investigation by a children's psychiatrist showed he could possibly suffer a form of autism. We were advised to send him to a medical-day-nursery. Meanwhile we also had video home training because Thomas had tantrums, asked for much negative attention and was insensitive to punishment.

Ultimately we decided to send him to a regular primary day school, however some troubles occurred with arithmetic and Dutch language. He did not communicate with teachers. In his fourth year he did not get his grades and had to redo the year.

Again tests were made and it occurred Thomas had an IQ of 65, an enormous fear of failure and a negative idea of himself. A children's psychologist diagnosed him with autism spectrum disease. The teachers saw loads of problems coming up, especially in class seven and eight, as he then was supposed to be more independent.

He had made enough friends; contact with them was normal although the friends always had to start the communication. Any joke was difficult to understand for him and usually caused trouble.

In 2006 we read an article on Dr. Tinus Smits, went to visit him and heard about the therapy for our son. Apart from homeopathic medicines like Carcinosinum and Saccharum officinale our Thomas takes daily doses of vitamin C and fish oil. From that moment on we got a totally new child. First of all his school results got much better. This was excellent for his self-confidence. The eczema he had all his life (back of the knees, arms, earlobes, cracks in the corners of the mouth) disappeared like snow in the sun. We now recognised this to be emotional problems.

In the last class of the primary school (age 12) he scored the national average standard. Thomas is now at a school where he gets extra help, but next year he will pass at a higher level of school without special support, because his results are 70% or higher. He looks and sounds OK, is planning and doing his homework all by himself. He has nice friends, is very social, takes others into account and has a good sense of humour. As target he wants to be a vet later and is studying hard.

Signed by two very happy and proud parents with sincere thanks to Dr. Tinus Smits

I have tried to give in this chapter an overview of how homeopathy — mainly Isotherapy — can nicely heal autism. To make the treatment clear and straight forward, I have taught all CEASE therapists to make a logical treatment plan based on the complete medical history of the child and the parents, without being distracted by different reactions and previous homeopathic remedies. Once all causative factors have been carefully resolved with Isotherapy, then classical or Inspiring Homeopathy can be used if necessary to give the finishing touch to the cure. This approach is much more pragmatic, can be easily understood by the parents, and gives reliably good results. The CEASE therapy should work in all cases, as long as the vital information is available. Fortunately as the CEASE therapy is under development, we are discovering more and more causative factors, thereby increasing still further the likelihood of complete cure.

CHAPTER 11

A RESPONSE TO DR. PAUL OFFIT'S BOOK:
AUTISM'S FALSE PROPHETS

First I want to thank Paul A. Offit for his book, which purports to prove scientifically that autism is not linked to vaccinations, because it actually confirms that I am on the right track. For example, he cites research comparing the effect of vaccines preserved with thimerosal (mercury) versus vaccines preserved with another neurotoxin, aluminum(hydr) oxide. Children vaccinated with both types have the same rate of autism, and Offit incorrectly concludes that vaccination is not the culprit. Instead, this research supports what I maintain in this book: that there are multiple causative factors, with mercury being only one of them. In fact I cite in this book the case of an autistic child who had never had any vaccinations but whose autism was cured only with the detoxification of his prenatal exposure to his mother's smoking and medications.

Paul Offit gives a different explanation for the cause of autism: genetics. But then how is it possible that autism has increased so dramatically in the last decades? A genetic disease can only increase 3 to 4% in a generation (30 years). Instead we need to look at epigenetics, the factors that can switch a gene on or off during a person's lifetime. Apparently there are many conditions in our modern life that can switch on the genes for autism, and that is the entire focus of my therapy. How to switch these genes off again? Most people, including most medical doctors, believe that genetic diseases are incurable. Certainly that is true of some genetic diseases like Down's syndrome, Duchenne, and many others.

But in autism there are real cures, which Paul Offit denies in his book. He claims that such cures are just temporary, and that shifts in the behavior of autistic children are common. The cases in this book are convincing evidence otherwise. A real scientist is interested in cases which contradict his beliefs, because they are what can lead to the discovery of something completely new.

Offit presents himself as a skeptic who only accepts what is scientifically proven. But reality is not limited to what science has proven. Science is not reality, it is just a perception of reality. The earth was round even while scientists believed it to be flat. Homeopathy has already been curing people for 200 years, demonstrated by clinical research, even though science still has no explanation for how it works. Homeopathy's healing power is a reality even though scientists who cannot explain it try to deny that it works. But this is backwards: it is the job of scientists to explain reality, not to deny reality based on their limited science. Scientists cannot be limited by their beliefs or by their self-interest, whether money or fame. Paul Offit, by the way, is the co-inventor of the rotavirus vaccine, although he has stated that he no longer profits from it.

Paul Offit has his own beliefs, as manifested in his book. He is entitled to his beliefs but not to claim that they are truth. He gives us a nice example. A mother feels that her son, on the other side of the world, has burned his arm. Offit calls it coincidence, but he is apparently unaware of the extensive research documenting such extrasensory phenomena, much of it conducted by the American government. This research is summarized in Lynn McTaggart's *The Field* and by the documentary *The Living Matrix*, a film by Greg Becker and Harry Massey

Paul Offit also disbelieves in alternative medicine, but he seems confused about what it is. He lumps together every therapy not applied in conventional medicine. Alternative medicine is non-toxic and stimulates the vital energy to engage in a healing process. This is in contrast to conventional medicine, which suppresses symptoms with mostly toxic products. It is not fair to focus on the dangers of alternative medicine, when more than 100,000 Americans die each year because of conventional medicine. This is the official number reported but is only the tip of the iceberg. In reality the total number of deaths from medical interventions is much higher. According to the *Journal of the American Medical Association (JAMA)*, medical treatment has become the third-leading cause of death after heart disease and cancer in the United States. (JAMA, July 26,2000;284(4):483-5) It is not alternative medicine that is dangerous, but conventional medicine. Maybe the most amazing point is that mainstream doctors, en masse, don't question their system's principle approach, which is primarily to suppress disease symptoms instead of healing them. One of the first principles in homeopathy, written down by its founder Dr. Samuel Hahnemann 200 years ago, is *primum non nocere*, 'first do no harm' — the same as the first principle of the Hippocratic Oath that regular doctors take.

Now let us study carefully the core of his book, which aims to prove that thimerosal and the measles vaccine are not the cause of autism. He succeeds brilliantly in this mission — and supports my own clinical experience that *mercury and the MMR cannot be the only or even the major cause of autism.* Amazingly, the whole discussion in the US has been focused only on mercury and not on vaccines in general. But in my experience, there is no difference between thimerosal- and aluminum-containing vaccines.

And here, with all due respect for his 'scientific' approach, Paul Offit makes a major error. Strictly, research has only proven that there is no difference in the number of autistic children when comparing vaccines with and without thimerosal. But that does not prove that vaccines do not cause autism! Offit states repeatedly that there is overwhelming evidence that vaccines do not cause autism, but that is an enormous overstatement of the research. There is no scientific research that has compared rates of autism in unvaccinated children with children receiving each one of the many childhood vaccines. So then how can a general statement be made that vaccines do not cause autism? Individual researchers have made this same mistake. Let us have a closer look at one of the sixteen research studies selected by Paul Offit to prove that vaccines do not cause autism.

A Hviid et al. Association between thiomersal-containing vaccine and autism. *JAMA* 2003 290: 1763-1766. The conclusion of their research: Thimerosal is not linked to autism. Their comment is as follows: 'What we have here is a superb study of what was, in effect, a real world before-after experiment. The study was huge, and comprehensive, covering almost 99% of children born in Denmark during a period during which a switch was made from use of a vaccine containing thimerosal to one that did not. It was the only vaccine given to children that did contain thimerosal. Moreover, diagnosis of autism or autistic spectrum disorder was according to strict criteria, and comprehensively applied. Follow up was for a minimum of four years, ensuring that almost all cases likely to occur should have occurred during that time. What we have, though, is powerful evidence that autism and autistic spectrum disorders do not arise from use of thimerosal in vaccines.'

Is this high standard research with undeniable results? The control group got vaccines preserved with another neurotoxic substance, aluminum(hydr)oxid. The only conclusion that can be drawn from this research is that both substances are equally likely to cause autism. And that is not all! A genuine researcher would even say that one of the other numerous potentially toxic substances in both vaccines is also to blame.

In irreproachable research, vaccinated children should be compared with unvaccinated children. In his prologue Paul Offit states that since the late 1990s, many studies have shown that the rates of autism are the same in vaccinated and unvaccinated children, so the notion that vaccines cause autism isn't a medical controversy. Apparently he is not clear about the definition of unvaccinated children. The following research gives us a perfect example.

Hviid et al. Childhood Vaccination and Nontargeted Infectious Disease Hospitalization. *JAMA* 2005;294:699-705. This research is currently used as scientific proof that vaccines are not undermining the immune system. Their definition of the control group is as follows: 'The unvaccinated group was primarily composed of children vaccinated with other vaccines.'

Dr. Hans Rümke, pediatrician and epidemiologist in Holland involved in the propagation of the vaccine program explains this failure to use real unvaccinated children in the control group as follows: 'Some years ago I have led research with the vaccination against the meningococ-C. The control group was given a Hepatitis B vaccination. That is the best research you can imagine.'

On page 109 Paul Offit presents the research of Eric Fombonne, which makes the same error: 'Obviously, removing thimerosal hadn't caused the increase [of autism].' Then Eric Fombonne writes: 'Parents of autistic children should be reassured that autism did not occur through immunizations.' Again the same generalization, even though the research covered only the thimerosal in vaccines, not the vaccines in general. Apparently Paul Offit also adopts Fombonne's explanation for the increase in autism: 'Factors accounting for the increase include a broadening of diagnostic concepts and criteria, increased awareness and, therefore, better identification of children with [autism] and improved access to services.' In other words he claims that there is no increase in the actual number of autistic children, inappropriately stepping out of his objective role as researcher to give his own personal opinions.

But what happens when we compare vaccinated children with a control group of truly unvaccinated children? Not surprisingly, this research is omitted from Paul Offit's book.

Kristensen/Aaby/Jensen BMJ 2000; 321:1435: Routine vaccinations and child survival: follow up study in Guinea-Bissau, West Africa. Methodologically correct, published with the full approval of the WHO in the *British Medical Journal*. Vaccinated children compared with *real* unvaccinated children. Conclusion: Vaccinated children between 0-1 year old have twice the risk of dying after the DTPP vaccination than unvaccinated children!

What to think about the Japanese experience in the seventies?
Cherry et al. 1988. *Pediatrics*, vol 81, no.6 part 2; p.939-984. Japan stopped vaccinating children under 2 years in 1975. This resulted in Japan having the lowest infant mortality rate in the world, whereas previously it had been in seventeenth place. The death rate due to neurological complications dropped from 37 in the preceding 5 year period to 3 in the 5 year period without DTP, while severe neurological complications with sequelae dropped from 57 to 8 in the same time periods.

And why does Paul Offit fail to mention Generation Rescue's survey published in 2007, entitled: *Vaccinated Children Two And A Half Times More Likely To Have Neurological Disorders Like ADHD And Autism, New Survey In California And Oregon Finds*. Although it is not a controlled study, the survey gives enough interesting results to at least stimulate questions for a scientist. For me, it exactly confirms my clinical findings.

Sadly enough there is no diagnostic tool in regular medicine to diagnose vaccination damage. If a child regresses a few days after his MMR shot and is eventually diagnosed autistic, there is no way to prove whether the regression was caused by the MMR. Therefore most family doctors and pediatricians prefer to stay on the safe side and deny any connection. It is a fact that many thousands of children regress to the point of autism shortly after the MMR, even sometimes within 24 to 48 hours. Why does Paul Offit not show any intellectual curiosity as to why? Personally I am not surprised that so many parents are convinced that the MMR is at fault.

And why not have intellectual curiosity about the findings of homeopathy? Here we have hundreds of cured or nearly cured cases, or cases well on the way to cure. In Isotherapy we have the perfect tool to discover a causal relationship between a vaccine or other substance and the regression to autism. If we suspect for example the MMR vaccine and we give the child homeopathically-prepared MMR in different potencies to detoxify the vaccine, then if there is no improvement the MMR was not involved. But if on the other hand the child clearly starts to heal, the conclusion (diagnosis) is that the MMR shot has substantially contributed to the genesis of his autism.

Through 300 cases I have come to the conclusion that most autistic children have not just one causative factor and that autism is a cumulative disease of different factors. In the great majority of my cases vaccinations are also involved, but that does not mean that vaccination is the only causation. Most of these children started already at an early age to have infections or other medical problems. They got antibiotics, anesthetics, antacids, anti-emetics, etc. The more medication in the first two years the greater the chance the child will become autistic. That is also true for the period of pregnancy and during delivery. The more medication the mother took, the greater the chance of having an autistic child. I have seen frequently that the way to autism was already prepared during the pregnancy and sometimes even before. Autism is in my experience a typical cumulative disorder which has to be healed by the elimination of all the causations that have contributed to its development. By clinical experience I have found out already that all vaccines can contribute to the development of autism, but also substances as xylometazolin (common nasal spray), antibiotics, anti epileptics, antacids, smoking, anesthesia, and possibly others that are still under investigation, including aspartame, glutamate, phthalates and Bisphenol A.

Paul Offit's book is an nice example of how scientific research can be (mis)used to prove your own beliefs or to serve the interests of the industry. There are so many ways to manipulate research and so many possibilities of selecting research that almost everything can be proven scientifically if the interest is great enough. His book does not honor true scientific research nor does it help to resolve the scourge of autism. Moreover it gives parents who strongly believe that vaccinations are involved in the disease of their child an undeserved feeling of guilt and incomprehension.

As in all fields of our human interaction, working together will give the best and fastest results. That is surely true for medicine. Nowadays still so many people suffer because of the artificial split between conventional and alternative medicine. Paul Offit's book has unfortunately not contributed to a better understanding between these two medicines and is rather a step backward in the understanding and solution of autistic disorders.

CHAPTER 12

WHAT CAN PARENTS THEMSELVES DO
TO HELP THEIR CHILD?

Avoid environmental factors to the extent possible in order to bypass genetic susceptibility

1. Give your child the best nutrition available, i.e., fresh organic foods, while avoiding packaged foods. By doing this you will prevent further toxicity from heavy metals, pesticides, flavor enhancers like MSG (glutamate), artificial sweeteners, color additives, GMOs, preservatives and other waste products. Many studies mentioned in John Erb's book, *The Slow Poisoning of America,* link MSG to obesity, diabetes, migraines and headaches, autism, ADHD, and even Alzheimer's.

2. Give your child sourdough bread instead of yeast bread to prevent the binding of zinc and magnesium to an insoluble complex with phytine acid and to enable the assimilation of nutritional zinc and magnesium. Since whole wheat sourdough bread is often very heavy, it would be better to start with lighter bread.

3. Give your child enough pure water without copper or other toxins.

4. Avoid the use of microwaves for all food and drinks; avoid also as much as possible plastic containers and packages.

5. Avoid as much as possible sugar, sweets in general and artificial sweeteners. They are poisonous to the intestines and pancreas and

several other tissues. Sugar also inhibits the production of EPA and DHA, both omega-3 fatty acids that are of crucial importance to the brain tissue.

6. Provide a quiet and peaceful environment for your child, eliminating excess stimuli such as TV, Game Boys or computers. Try to really be there for your child.

7. Make sure your child is well grounded to the earth. Static electricity may give rise to both emotional/mental disorders and physical complaints. Synthetic clothing, isolating shoes (rubber or plastic soles) and synthetic floor coverings (vinyl) should therefore be avoided. Even wooden floors with a thin plastic covering can be harmful. Have your child walk around barefoot at home, and barefoot on the grass or earth as much as possible, if the environment is safe. Eliminate all electric appliances in the bedroom such as electric alarm clocks, TV, computers, cell phones (mobiles) or audio equipment.

8. Provide a healthy sleeping environment for your child. A healthy bed should not contain any metal, because it reinforces the magnetic disturbances of the earth and of the man-made electro-magnetic environment. If possible, have your child sleep facing north or east to align with the magnetic field of the earth which goes from the South Pole to the North Pole. Stop using babyphones and phones with DECT technology (most wireless (baby)phones), they give a very strong radiation field. A dark room is important for the production of melatonin (sleep hormone).

9. Avoid antibiotics since they impair intestinal flora and consequently increase underlying problems. In case of infection, opt for naturopathic solutions. In case medical treatment is necessary for your child, try to find energetic solutions such as homeopathy which boost the immune system, instead of symptomatic treat-

ments that are suppressive. If your child is apparently not functioning well on the mental, emotional or physical level, e.g. has a chronic runny nose or repeated other infections, is easily tired, cross, has bad appetite and is not sleeping well, do not wait until he gets sick and needs another course of antibiotics, but have him treated preventively by natural medicine. If you suppress symptoms with regular medicine, the disturbed energy will remain, and sooner or later it will cause the same or deeper health problems.

10. Do not vaccinate your child any further; your son or daughter is probably already in bad health because of the shots; do not add to this but seek help and healing first.

Add nutrients to maximize your child's health

11. Put your child on omega-3 fatty acids, the highest and purest quality you can find. Normally I prescribe not more than 500mg a day. Avoid the overconsumption of omega-6 fatty acids from soy and corn, which are mainly in processed food. Omega-3 fatty acids are anti-inflammatory, omega-6 are pro-inflammatory. The ideal ratio would be 1:1, but modern food contains 1:25!

12. Administer the two different vitamins Cs yourself. Both are available in tablets or capsules and as powder. The maximum dose is determined by the 'bowel tolerance test': gradually increase the dose until diarrhea appears, then the dose should be lowered a little bit until it disappears. This slightly lower dose is the correct amount and is completely safe; only patients with hemochromatosis should avoid extra vitamin C, because vitamin C stimulates iron absorption. But you don't have to give the 'maximum dose'. The general rule is not more than 1000mg per year of age. So a child of four years can be given 4000mg a day divided over three doses a day. That means three times an ascorbate of 1000mg and 3

times ascorbyl palmitate of 500mg (each tablet contains 200mg of vitamin C). That makes 3600mg per day. At 6 years and older the maximum dose I advise is still 6 grams a day, which is generally enough to attain our goal.

13. Give extra zinc: 10mg for children under 4, 20mg from 4 to 8, and 30mg for 9 years and older.

Then make an appointment with a CEASE therapist. Autism is a serious disease that can be treated successfully, but even though I have given you a lot of information about its treatment in this book, it needs professional help. Otherwise you will ultimately be disappointed and not get the results you hoped to achieve. Your child is too precious to treat yourself.

CHAPTER 13

PARENTS' TESTIMONIALS

Testimonial of Joost's mother

On a beautiful summer day the most wonderful thing happened to me: I found out I was pregnant! In the months to come I read all the books on pregnancy available in shops and libraries. The last book I came across was on a very special autistic boy. I never finished the book because during the last chapter I went into labor and I never got to the last page because my son was born.

From that last page I read, I could start my own book of my search in a world of hope and despair, understanding and misunderstanding.

My son was born on the first of March, a healthy baby, a miracle, my life was a pink cloud. Although he cried considerably, he developed well, laughed at six weeks, crawled at nine months, walked at 13 months and babbled cheerfully. He preferred to be outside, walking in the forest or going out with mummy and daddy.

One outing I will never forget, taking him to the playground. That does not sound special, does it? However there I met a mother of a boy just a bit older than mine. She told me her son had always been healthy like mine but that all had changed after the MMR shot. He did not make contact anymore, cried a lot, started to babble like a baby again, and withdrew into his own world.

I thought then just for a minute about the MMR my son would get in two weeks, but doesn't everyone have their child vaccinated? That would not happen to us... is what I unfortunately thought.

Yes... and then... also for us... the huge change in *his* but also in *our* lives. The day of the MMR stays indelibly stamped in my memory. It was as if my dear little son already knew what was going to happen to him, as if his future had been decided already.

He shrieked as he had never done before, he resisted so hard that two doctors came to hold him. I held my own child down so they could give him the shot. I really believe that in that moment he lost faith in the world and partly also in me.

A week later the misery started. He withdrew more and more into his own (fantasy) world, making less and less eye contact. He had many ear infections. All toys making noise made him put his hands on his ears and shriek loudly.

At two he hardly played with toys anymore. He could sit for hours on the couch listening to quiet music. When driving, I often glanced to see whether I had forgotten to take him with me he was so quiet. He was locked into his own world.

Kindergarten was a drama... I brought him a few times with his knees trembling. However he did nothing there, did not play with the other kids. He only watched. This was too much for my 'motherly feelings' and after two months I removed him from the kindergarten.

In the first year of primary school, when he was four, nothing had changed. He could only go to school in the morning because he was oversensitive to all the stimuli. He had very few friends, hardly participated in any activity, instead retired into his own world.

Because his health was also deteriorating, I decided to go to an iridologist with whom I had had good results. His tests showed that my son's health problems could not be put right until the MMR shot was detoxified. Many things had gone wrong from the MMR and the poison in his body had to be eliminated. He referred us to Dr. Tinus Smits and that proved to be the turnabout from despair to hope and from incomprehension to complete understanding.

We became alive again when we heard that complete recovery would be possible. Not only he became alive again, but also we, over a period of three years.

It all started after the first series of MMR detoxification. We were asked to come and talk to his second grade teacher. Something had happened that she could not explain. My little son who normally was on his own, now suddenly was in the centre of attention of the tough boys. He really was very present. He talked too much, was naughty during lessons, lifted other children to show off how strong he was... and even quarrelled. Many a parent would not have liked such a conversation with the teacher but I was very delighted without expressing it clearly to the teacher. All of a sudden my child was making a lot of contact with others, even though maybe not always in the right way.

After the next detoxification series, more of his lost qualities emerged again. His eye contact was improving. At school he started joining group activities, however he still would not let anyone other than a family member touch him. So holding hands while singing and lice inspections by other mothers were still dramatic. His sheer endless fantasy world where he could bring alive anything he observed in his surroundings, was still a point of special interest.

And then there were still his multiple obsessions: for the brand names of all the soft drink bottles, his obsession for waterfalls, for the names of all countries in the world (at six years old), for number work ... there was still good detoxification to be done.

So we continued the detoxification process with Dr. Tinus Smits, clearing the DTPP and the Neisvac-C. Often he had violent reactions during this process. After taking those tiny pills, my little son could weep distressingly as if he wanted to throw out all the sorrow of the whole world.

Sometimes he could get so terribly angry with screaming or stamping his feet. I had never seen him like that before. Up till now all had remained locked up inside him.

By venting all that anger and sorrow, he was able to show more and more of his feelings. Little by little he started living in the real world, leaving his fantasy world behind. We could have conversations about the real world and not the world of teddy bears and other cuddly toys anymore.

After further series of detoxification, he brought more and more friends home with him, and he got a number of invitations for parties too. For most parents this was quite normal, but for me still so meaningful. We had found the right way.

We are not yet quite there as he still has a few obsessions. However we now have a great kid who loves family parties, makes his class laugh with his jokes, talks constantly from 8 in the morning until 8 at night, and who yesterday during a class trip addressed - in poetic form and standing on a litter basket - the crowd waiting in rows to be admitted into an attraction.

Tinus Smits, for me you are a hero, who brought life back to my son, to me and to my husband.

Thank you!

Testimonial of Margriet's parents

In June 2007 when our daughter Margriet was 7 years old, we started with a sugar free diet, organic food as much as possible, vitamins and Saccharum off. 30C. She was diagnosed with ADHD, PDD-NOS, and was a most obstinate girl whom we could not manage. Visiting other people with her was a real affliction. People did not like us to come over, so most of time we stayed home so as not to bother our friends. Margriet had almost always diarrhea, could not eat normally, ate very little, and took an hour and a half for dinner. She drank large quantities and loved anything sweet. She ate only two types of vegetables and two types of meat, and those just in small amounts. As a consequence she was very thin.

After three weeks of treatment by Dr. Tinus Smits, the change was unbelievable. That day we ate fried fish (I would always put everything on her plate that I had cooked for ourselves). Margriet ate the fish and looked at me in amazement. "Mom, I don't understand, I can put this in my mouth, swallow it and eat it, how is that possible?" From that moment she started to eat everything and at a normal rate. Now two years later she even eats food other kids usually don't like. She now asks regularly when we are going to eat because she is hungry.

After this first treatment Dr. Smits started with the detox of methyldopa, a high blood pressure medication I used during my pregnancy. Margriet reacts quite violently to these courses of detoxification. She has a difficult time and we as parents did too, but we have been doing them on and off for more than a year now. Her reactions grow less and less each time, but we want to keep repeating them, because after each one we notice progress in her behavior. On the social level Margriet has improved substantially. She now has a 'best friend'.

After the detoxification of the methyldopa we are starting with the clearance of her vaccines.
I would like to recommend such an approach to all parents, no matter

what the rest of the world says and do not give up! It is great to see your child improve in this way.

Testimonial of Rob's parents

We would like to share our story because our lives changed quite a lot when Dr. Tinus Smits started treating our son.

Rob had his first vaccinations at the age of 10 weeks while suffering from a cold and the second series shortly afterwards as we had to move to Canada. The health centre told us that it was standard procedure.

At this young age he always had a cold (a running nose and drooling), smelly watery stool, never slept in one stretch during the night, and cried often. He never obeyed and he reacted badly to people around him.

At age three and a half he had his tonsils and adenoids taken out and tubes put in his ears. We expected that he would be much better now, but there was hardly any change.

When going to school (4 years old) he appeared to be 'different', he was tested and diagnosed as PDD-NOS.

Because his sister had celiac disease and we were searching for a relation between the two illnesses (a cousin was in the same situation) we found the site of Tinus Smits by chance.

Dr. Smits started his series of detoxification step by step – vaccinations, anesthetics, antibiotics, parents' vaccinations – and consequently Rob has now become a completely different child.

He is 10 now. The most important thing is that he is manageable now and that he engages in mutual contact. Also his grandparents and teachers at school are amazed. He has friends now, his results at school are good and at home with his sisters the ambiance has changed.

I myself, his mother, was on the verge of a nose operation. Dr. Smits advised me to take a series of homeopathic diluted pollens and mites (glycyphagus), and my nose and sinuses have been clear for two years, no blocked nose or sinusitis any more.

We are very grateful to Dr. Smits for what he did for us. We as parents know his art of working and healing really helps. We therefore hope many will continue his good work.

Testimonial of Yarnick's parents

I would like to tell you what Dr. Smits meant for our son Yarnick and for us.

Until he was a year and a half his development was normal, we had eye contact, he reacted normally to us, could be consoled, etc. He was a happy and sweet little boy. But from the age of 18 months we were hardly able to make contact with him any more. He had numerous ear infections which were very difficult to heal, accompanied by a chronic flu. His speech got stuck at the level of a one year old.

When three years old, he finally got tubes in his ears after many courses of antibiotics. He was completely in his own world and incapable of social interaction, in spite of his good hearing. At first we had assumed Yarnick could not hear us and lagged in speech for that reason, however this appeared not to be the case.

His whole attitude changed and he became a frustrated boy. This behavior manifested itself as tantrums, headbanging, shrieking, biting, hyperactivity, refusing to fall asleep and never sleeping through till next morning, inability to be reprimanded, keeping his hands over his ears, strict rituals and great difficulty coping with changes in daily life.

When he was four and a half we took him to Dr. Smits, who started the detoxification of his vaccinations. Yarnick had heavy reactions, the ear infections came back temporarily together with vomiting, diarrhea and regressing into certain old patterns. He sometimes was terribly ill. However, after each detoxification we noticed an improvement in his behavior. Very shortly after the first course, he never got ill again (except during the detoxifications).

Now Yarnick is six and a half and his behavior has improved immensely. He still is under Dr. Smits' care to detoxify his father's vaccinations, a treatment to which he had again a violent reaction.

To date we have not completed all detoxifications, however we can already state that Yarnick improved enormously in his general behavior.

All the difficulties mentioned above have practically disappeared and also his speech has started to develop again. He is interested in other people around him and we have better contact with him.

To date we can conclude that the detoxification of the vaccines had a most positive result for Yarnick. As Yarnick now has more fun, is able to express himself much better and has less frustrations, our family-life has positively changed.

We are forever grateful to Dr. Smits.

Testimonial of Sem's parents

Sem was born by caesarean due to a breech presentation. He was an easy and happy baby till his ear problems started at 8 months. He got one ear infection after the other, so a lot of antibiotics. After one year Sem changed, it seemed like he did not hear well any more, while as a baby he reacted to all and everything.

Sem got tubes in his ears and then many hearing tests and examinations including an examination under anaesthesia. A cochlear loss of 30 to 40 dB was measured, indicating a substantial and permanent loss of hearing. He had to be fitted with a hearing aid.

However, as parents we thought something was not right here. We went to another hospital and the doctor there said immediately we should have Sem tested, that in his opinion Sem was autistic. Your world collapses at that moment, because autism is incurable according to conventional medicine.

However, once more I could not accept that our happy little boy had changed into a child that did not even react when his parents came home from work.

I started searching on the internet and luckily I found Dr. Tinus Smits' site.

We started immediately with fish oil and within two weeks he heard the planes flying over and looked up. Unbelievable!

Sem has been under CEASE therapy for two years now and a lot has changed already. Sem hears everything now without a hearing aid. He has been tested at the Centre for audiology: no hearing loss anymore!

The antibiotics, the anaesthesia, MMR and a tetanus shot given to me during pregnancy (this should never have happened), all this has been detoxified now.

Sem has become more alert, happier, and we have more eye contact. His comprehension has also improved. Right now we are detoxifying the DTPP, to Sem's great distress. Every time he has a high fever, turns inwardly again and has lots of tantrums.

This is the fifth course of DTPP and now slowly he is improving again. He gets naughty again and the twinkle in his eyes is returning.

Of course there were difficult moments, when he was falling back to old problems for months at a time. He had difficulties with those courses because they had to be repeated often and it did take a long time.

The fact that Sem still does not talk, does not make us any happier. Nor the reports of the psychologists who think they know all about your child. But no matter what, he is still improving and we have the fullest confidence in the therapy of Dr. Smits. We shall continue as long as it takes to get Sem to talk again and to be able to enjoy life as a capable person.

Testimonial of Wouter's parents

We want to share our experiences with other parents because so many things have changed for us and our son.

In November 2007 we came to Dr. Tinus Smits with our son Wouter, nine years old. He had been diagnosed with PDD-NOS. We were desperate as our G.P. advised us to put Wouter on regular medication, because he was very depressed.

In Dr. Smits' waiting room he was slouching in a chair, tired and flabby. When we entered into the consulting room, he made himself comfortable in a wicker chair, leaving his shoes behind. I thought immediately: Here we are in the right place. Wouter felt at ease, a beginning had been made. The diagnosis PDD-NOS did not give Dr. Smits much information, but he wanted to know everything about Wouter and his history.

In this way we found many important leads. The first little globules were prescribed and the vitamin C and fish oil were taken regularly. Thank goodness, Dr. Smits says no regular drugs while they are healing, which is also better because this type of overmedicated child could easily slip into drug abuse as a teenager, according to Dr. Smits.

Every few months we met, from time to time we phoned for some tips and advice. Dr. Smits was a good listener and always phoned back even very late at night.

A few weeks ago when we saw Dr. Smits, we went through all the complaints from day one. We realized that Wouter is about 80% cured. It is incredible when we think of all those complaints today. Dr. Smits has achieved a lot and with great courage we'll start the last 20% as he is not yet satisfied. We'll go to the maximum.

Dr. Smits, we are grateful that we met you. You are a very special person. We loved it each time, seeing you full of dedication behind your desk. Your big hands, your fountain pen, your notepaper. Kindest regards from all of us.

Testimonial of Arjen's parents

Our son Arjen is now 11 years old going into the eighth grade after summer vacation. He is doing well at school, he feels fine now; however that was not always the case. He has an extensive medical record.

It started with a difficult birth followed by breastfeeding problems because of his bad coordination. After a few weeks he also got intestinal problems, with blood and mucus in his stool and diarrhea. This lasted until he was 18 months old. He had a weak immune system and was ill very often.

Then he reacted more violently at each vaccination. The vaccination to be given at 11 months was postponed to 15 months. After that one our problems really started. After the first violent reactions, his stool became worse and he got attacks which looked like epileptic seizures. He became hyperactive and had problems with making contact. We did not dare to visit other people as he threw everything he could get his hands on, even against windows and TV. His mental development remained at the age of his last vaccination at 15 months. Now at the age of 18 months, he was 6 months behind.

The result of all this was that we were referred to several specialists, the child-neurologist, child-psychiatrist, and child-gastro-enterologist, which resulted in placing him in a medical day-care centre.

In the long run what really helped was the alternative medicine. At first Arjen started to improve with the orthomanual naturopathic doctor, but unfortunately this doctor retired and we had to find somebody else.

Finally, after a thorough research, we found Dr. Smits and a good osteopath. Then his digestive problems, his hyperactivity, immune system and concentration improved more and more.

As a result – after three years of medical day-care – he was allowed into a regular school, into second grade! We were over the moon; this was what we hoped for. The tests showed an average intelligence however socially still weak. The latter would disappear completely over the coming years.

His social emotional development now is normal for his age. Arjen is spontaneous and social with a strong will. His school results are above average. All this makes us as parents most happy and very proud.

All this has been quite a long path to take. Fortunately we found the right doctors and therapists when we needed them.

Testimonial of Seo's grandparents followed by the testimonial of his mother
One page is far too short to express our enthusiasm for this treatment. A lengthy trilogy would be more appropriate. Once you enter the world of autism and you are confronted with all the misery which this disorder provokes, you are closer to tears than to laughter. The worst is that you know that there is a way out. But when you talk about it with people, you find an enormous prejudice about homeopathy. We are guilty of that ourselves. Before we had experienced the results of this therapy closely, we were burdened with quite a lot of skepticism. But since we know that this therapy really pays off, it proves to be so difficult to convince other parents to follow this treatment. It is heartbreaking to see that Seo's classmates make no or very little progress. Even though all parents know that we apply this treatment, there is nobody who dares to take that step.

The birth of a grandchild is one of the milestones in life that gives intense joy. A dream that after 16 months would change into a nightmare. From one moment to the next, the day after a particular vaccination, all life disappeared from our Seo. All knowledge and progress that he had made in his early life had suddenly disappeared. His first words and his contact with his parents, grandparents and everybody who loved him was disrupted abruptly. What remained was an apathetic child with lifeless eyes and a far-away look, who had lost all connection with reality.

Then started a long journey to diagnostic centers and specialists. The results were devastating: autism in the first degree. This disorder means an enormous burden for everybody, not only for the child but also for everyone around him: lack of contact, enormous outbursts of anger, problems with eating and toilet-training, etc., etc. We had already resigned ourselves to the idea that our grandson would face a difficult future. Nevertheless grandma did not throw in the towel. She has read tons of books and spent many nights combing the internet searching for answers. During one of her searches she found your website, the first site where possible help could be given. Honestly I have to admit that personally I was very skeptical towards homeopathy. Happily my wife stood her ground.

The result was that we soon went to see Dr. Smits with our daughter and Seo, a day that would become a real turnabout. The detox courses which Seo is still continuing have caused a wonderful reversal. To be honest, it is not a path strewn with roses. The detox reactions are sometimes so frightening that doubts come up whether you want to continue. But the reward for our perseverance was always in relation to the detox reactions. The worse the reactions, the greater the progress. It happened more than once that Seo was catapulted two years back in time. In the morning all life would seem to have disappeared from the child and in the afternoon, almost from one moment to another, a kind of awakening took place with a spectacular progress. It is almost an endless task to give examples. Nevertheless I want to describe some amazing events.

Seo had a tricycle, but he could not master the dynamics of bicycling.

The second day after the administration of a high potency of a detox remedy he is coming home from school, looks at us and says: 'Seo will go bicycling.' He goes to the garden, climbs up his tricycle and starts to pedal around as if he has done this already for years.

Another peculiar event. We have tried with almost infinite patience to teach Seo to count, but without success. It simply did not work. He did not even try to repeat the numbers. One day he had to go to the family doctor to take care of a cut that he got falling down. The doctor's office had a chart with numbers and letters to test vision. Seo stood up from his chair, approached the chart and pointed with his finger to the numbers, pronouncing clearly the numbers from 1 to 10 correctly.

One more amazing incident is the following anecdote. In our free time we write columns for a major pigeon racing magazine. One day we were writing a story on our computer. Seo came and stood next to us and looked at the screen. 'That's a lot of letters, grandpa', he said with admiration. I answered: 'When you grow up you will be able to do this too.' He looked at me pensively and asked: "Seo try also?" Two days later he knew all the letters of the alphabet and was able to type words of 3 or 4 letters. He had not learned the ABC, but the QWERTY as arranged on the keyboard.

I could describe dozens of examples of such surprising events. No, all problems are far from completely gone. On the social level and with his motor skills there are still serious problems. But we are actually after two and a half years only halfway through the detoxification process, and the results are already a thousand times better than we could have hoped in our wildest dreams. We are absolutely convinced that our Seo after the complete treatment will be able to function well in our sometimes very complicated society. As an originally absolute non-believer I would like to advise everybody to follow this CEASE therapy. Complete healing will be perhaps not always possible, but every progress already means a world of difference for these children and their environment. You can be sure, this really works!!

Testimonial of Seo's mother
As my parents have described, many things have changed in our life since we started the detox courses with our son Seo. My parents have been closely involved from the beginning in the ups and downs of my son because of special circumstances. As already stated everything went wrong from the time he was 16 months old, one day after a vaccination. Finally when a speech delay became more and more evident, I went to the family doctor, but he told me that this happens frequently especially in boys. It is your first child and you don't have much experience with small children, the doctor said.

Six months later we took him for a hearing test thinking he might not hear well ... but that was not the problem. After that he spent two weeks in a children's psychiatric center for observation. There the diagnosis of autism was made. He had many typical autistic behavioral patterns such as spinning, walking on his tiptoes and flapping.

Together with the home care we have looked for a special school, and from the age of three he could go to school. But the year was not very fruitful, there was hardly any progress. He was completely in his own world.

The visit to Dr. Smits brought a turnaround in Seo's life. We are now half way through the detox process and even if it was not always easy, we noticed great progress. The babbling changed to clear sounds, then short syllables and sometimes you could even understand a word if you listened with full attention. And then suddenly the big moment was there, he said: 'Mommy' and that was the beginning of an enormous development in speech and language. Now he is able to express himself well and he makes beautiful sentences; he also understands what you ask him. He became potty-trained and is able to enjoy his play. He even is so intelligent that he makes jokes with us. Then he says: 'this is a joke, hahaha...' He has a good memory and often tells stories about the past when he was 'small.' He then says: 'When I was a little baby ...…..' He also enjoys being cuddled and he also cuddles with me sometimes spontaneously.

Now half way through the treatment I am very happy with the results, our life has become a lot easier and more pleasant. Of course I hope he will heal completely with the remaining treatment and that many children will be helped with this method.

CHAPTER 14

SUCCESSFUL CASE REPORTS OF CEASE THERAPISTS

During the recent five-day CEASE training course in Holland, I noticed that some participants who were very advanced homeopaths were already applying the principles of detoxifying causations from my earlier seminars. They told the audience wonderful experiences and excellent cases. Then I thought of asking them to write case reports also. Here they are! It is amazing to see how this approach can resolve so much suffering among children and their parents. Hopefully a few of these case reports will demonstrate that others can use this method successfully. Every homeopath who applies these principles correctly will get the same results.

Case report from Wil Meijer-Kal, CEASE therapist at Bennebroek, the Netherlands. Case of successful detoxification of vaccines
I saw Tommy in June 2000, age 3 years and 9 months, a beautiful boy with curly blond hair. When he walked into my room I had the immediate feeling: 'What went wrong with this boy?'

CEASE therapy wasn't available yet, but I practiced the detoxification method from Tinus Smits' earlier teachings.

The first 15 months of his life he developed well, physically and mentally. Then he got a convulsion from high fever. In the two weeks after the convulsion, Tommy's behavior changed drastically. He became aggressive, hit everyone who came near, banged his head, shouted and screamed and could only make groaning noises. He did not speak. He liked to cuddle with his mother and clearly regressed to an infantile state.

In spite of this convulsion Tommy was given the MMR vaccination two weeks later!

When I saw him for the first time, he had a very high pain treshhold, was very strong, showed a lot of aggression and hit himself. Rituals were important to him and if things didn't follow through according to his rituals he yelled and became aggressive. He spoke with much difficulty, just single words, and omitted the consonants at the beginning of a word. He was very fearful; he didn't want to go to sleep in his own bed and only felt safe with his mum and dad. He always hid behind his mother, didn't dare to be alone, and was afraid of the dark. He had panic attacks. When his mother managed to settle him down he was very timid and cuddled up with her.

Tommy was placed in a special school since July 1999. In school he did not want to do what he was told, he just sat there. He wanted to be out in the open air, to run around, but he saw no danger. He was fond of playing with water, loved to ride his tricycles and was crazy about cars. He liked everything that goes fast. He loved animals, wanted to touch them, but then he would kick them out of the blue.

When Tommy was hit by other children he did not defend himself, he just let it happen. In return he himself can show very annoying behavior, driving the family nuts. His older brother (9) was often the victim of Tommy's behavior.

Physically Tommy had asthma and needed an inhaler with Ventolin (1x) and Flixotide (3x). He had otitis media several times a year and had antibiotics at least 8 times already in his short life.

I decided to start with a series of the MMR vaccination in homeopathic preparation, planning giving him the DTPP/Hib series after that.

As a reaction on the detoxification of the MMR, Tommy became less aggressive and more relaxed, and he needed his Ventolin and Flixotide much less frequently. But in the third week he developed a hip infection and he could not walk for a whole week. He also complained about his knee. Then after a week he spontaneously started to walk again and the symptoms of the hip infection subsided.

I decided to repeat the MMR series until no reaction occurred.

Then Tommy went through a phase of having copious bowel movements. He developed a runny nose but it did not affect his lungs. He made definite progress in his speech.

I didn't see or hear from Tommy any more for more than a year. His mother spontaneously called me then to let me know that Tommy was developing so well that he was allowed to attend a regular school. He was able to quit the special school!

Then, four years later, I heard from her again (Tommy was 8 years and 8 months old at that point). He was still doing fine, his reading, writing and memory were all very good, and he was playing the drums in a brass band. He was tall and strong for his age, played judo and seemed relaxed.

When he was 13 years old, his mother informed me that he was in his first year of a technical school, took his homework seriously, loved to cook, and helped his mother in her flower shop.

He never forgets anything once he has mastered a skill. His motor activity however is giving him some trouble. He has friends to play with, but also can be on his own, doing the things he likes to do.

Tommy is doing fine!

Comments of Dr. Smits: This is an interesting case. It reveals something very important. Every doctor would have blamed his disease on his convulsions, but fever convulsions almost never cause permanent harm. Here clearly the MMR shot during his convalescence (too early!) has blocked the healing process that should have taken place after his convulsions. Once this blockage has been lifted by the detoxification of the MMR, Tommy was able to heal again. His vital energy was blocked, causing not only behavior problems, but also physical complaints like the many ear infections. Children should never be vaccinated when they are ill until they have completely recovered.

Case of shaken baby syndrome from Ton Jansen, CEASE therapist at Den Hoorn, the Netherlands.

I am personally convinced that in many of these cases vaccinations are involved and parents are unjustly blamed, even jailed, because their baby had a bad vaccine reaction. This horrible injustice will continue as long as vaccinations are not considered as possible causations.

Case of shaken-baby syndrome

Jordy was six months old when I saw him in my practice. The parents had lost their parental rights because they were accused of maltreating their little baby (shaken-baby syndrome). Shortly after the second vaccination Jordy became epileptic. A couple of days later he got a cerebral hemorrhage and was hospitalized. When he was discharged, the parents were required to always have a third person present because of a strong suspicion of shaken-baby-syndrome. Jordy's maternal grandmother was later allowed to care for the baby.

During this first consultation Jordy was in his mother's arms. His mouth was open, he was unable to swallow, and he was drip-fed by his nose. The parents and the grandmother were panicked.

The parents told me that their baby was completely healthy the first 2 months. He had shrieked after the first vaccination and was not well for a while. I prescribed the DTPP/Hib in different potencies in a short course of 15 days and then saw him again in my office. A miracle seemed to have happened. Jordy looked around, drank from his bottle, and often kept his mouth closed. His overall flabbiness seemed to have disappeared and his muscles were stronger. Sometimes he still swallowed the wrong way. I repeated the whole course and saw him again 4 weeks later. The healing process had continued and there were no longer any residual complaints. He was again a completely healthy child. The parents got their parental rights back after a year. The nightmare was over!

Case of treatment during pregnancy with anti-RhD globulin
Karina is a girl 6 months old and a very easy going child. She rarely cries, moves very little and does not turn around yet. She has a remarkable stiffness and seems to lack any desire to move. Her mother had an uncomplicated pregnancy and her delivery was easy lasting only two and a half hours. Her daughter weighed 3.7 kilograms (8 pounds).

However her mother is Rh negative and got an anti-RhD-globulin injection eight weeks before her delivery. That is why I chose to detoxify the anti-RhD globulin, each potency four times during a period of eight weeks. After this course her capacity of moving increased dramatically and her stiffness has gone completely.

Case of local anesthesia (artecain) during pregnancy
Kyra is a nine year old girl diagnosed with autism. The first time I saw her was the end of March, 2009.

Until six months she drank well from the bottle, but then she began to deteriorate and at seven months she was admitted to the hospital in dehydrated condition. Her mother had an extra-uterine pregnancy before she got pregnant with Kyra, which had to be removed by surgery.

Kyra did not have clear reactions to the vaccinations. She can't eat nor drink by herself and caring for her takes a lot of work. Until her fourth year she is drip-fed. She clearly has been stuck in her oral phase, she puts everything into her mouth, and she hates water.

I prescribe her a detoxifying course of DTTP/Hib and MMR, each potency four times. However the reactions are not convincing. I decide to repeat the course.

When I see her again in July, she eats bread again herself and has gained weight. Her speech and comprehension have improved, e.g. she now knows the difference between a horse and a cow. She wants to hug again. It seems like all has improved. So I repeat the course once more.

Then at the next consultation, after completion of the checklist her mother tells me that in the third month of her pregnancy she had a local anesthesia (artecain) for root canal work. This clarifies her daughter's actual problems. Probably this artecain has been the cause of Kyra's inability to function. The detoxification with artecain gives an unbelievable result. She now really looks at me, eats herself with a spoon or fork and is potty trained. Also emotionally Kyra has improved considerably; she now expresses her joy and does not hide her sadness or anger any more.

Her mother says she has improved 80% but I guess that this is a bit exaggerated. 50% would be a better assessment in my eyes. There is still a lot to be cleared.

We repeat the course again and with success. This gives again a considerable improvement. Now I agree with the 80% estimation of her mother. She is over the moon. With the third course of artecain we hope to heal Kyra completely.

Case report from Collette van Hardenbroek, CEASE therapist at Sassenheim, the Netherlands. Case of successful detoxification of different substances
Anton was 12 years old and diagnosed with Asperger's syndrome when I first saw him at my practice. His problems started from about six years. He was easily angered and would strike without hesitation. He did a special training in social skills, but it hardly changed anything. During a short time he used Ritalin because of his poor concentration, but he could only pay attention to something when he was really interested.

He took everything literally and was very sensitive to touch, immediately feeling attacked. He was highly intelligent with an excellent memory, although he had poor motor skills, disliking sports at school. He functioned better when everything was well structured. He loved playing checkers and computer games, reading, and looking at National Geographics.

As a child he was active and slept very lightly (the slightest noise woke him up). He was always hungry. He did not start speaking until he was two, but then he was a chatterbox. He was afraid outside of his home, and he found cars both very dangerous and irritating. He was also afraid of flies and in the dark.

He was easily irritated and felt better from hitting. He did not like to sleep late because he did not want to miss anything. He had a good relationship with his mother. He spent most of the day at his computer. He did not make eye contact easily.

After that first consultation I started to repertorize his symptoms as classical homeopaths usually do, but there were so many symptoms. Remedies like Mercurius, Bufo, Hyoscyamus, Zincum came up, but none of them felt like the right remedy. I had already learned about detoxifying vaccines with Tinus Smits, and because his mother had indicated herself that after the vaccination he did not want to sit on her lap any more, I decided to start with the DTPP. Anton did not have clear reactions during the detoxification itself, but afterwards he made considerable progress. His contact with others improved, he became more flexible, his fear of the dark disappeared and he started to eat better, even fruits. After a second course of DTPP he became more and more relaxed, but his sleep did not improve.

Then I detoxified the MMR, which resulted in his sleep problems disappearing along with his anxiety about going to a new secondary school. He also clearly showed more interest in people.

Anton did well in the first class of the secondary school. He had good contact with his classmates and was content to learn a lot of things. He was attentive and his anger had almost disappeared. He still had problems with his concentration.

Then I gave him Lycopodium LM1 and LM2 for several months. His marks improved and he felt more relaxed. He himself took care of everyday things and took on more responsibilities.

After another class with Tinus, I asked his mother what medications she got during the pregnancy and delivery, and what medications Anton got in early childhood. Quite a lot of medical drugs had been used: oxytocin to start the contractions, Neisvac-C, nasal spray (Xylomethazolin), fucidine crème, triamcinolon crème and aspirin. He was hypersensitive to aspartame and got diarrhea from it. I also discovered that I had not detoxified his Hib vaccination. So I continued his treatment with that one. Taking the 1M he got heavy headache with vomiting. When I asked his mother how far along the healing process was, she answered 60%.

After the CEASE course I repeated the MMR and DTPP detoxification once more in a short course. To his mother's amazement, he then spontaneously set the table in the morning, took out the dog, and cleaned his room on his own initiative.

During the detoxification of the aspartame he reacted with headaches and sat listless on the couch.

We still have not reached complete healing, but Anton and his mother are happy with what has been done so far. He talks to me directly and looks straight at me. I always laugh about his quick and associative thinking. It is nice to discover in this way the possibilities of the CEASE therapy.

CHAPTER 15

CONCLUSION

In this book I have attempted to give as much information as possible to the parents of autistic children and to all those who are interested in or concerned with the treatment of children with autism and behavior disorders. Many case examples show how well Isotherapy works while directly rebalancing the damaged energy. This therapy also gives valuable and reliable information about the different causations which lead to autism and other profound development problems in our children. Certainly there is still more to be discovered, but at this point we can say that the majority of causative factors have already been identified. Within a few years there will be CEASE therapists all over the world, and the collection of data — especially concerning causative factors — will increase enormously.

The duration of CEASE therapy is still a concern, with most cases taking two or three years and even longer. Soon with many CEASE therapists working together, we will search for ways to shorten the process to one or two years. The development of CEASE therapy so far has been limited to my own work as an individual for the past several years.

I realize that there is still no scientific proof for the effectiveness of this therapy, but fortunately parents do not have to wait for proof to try it for their child. However, to make this therapy well established as a powerful tool for healing autism, this research is necessary and has already been undertaken by the CEASE organization.

In the coming years our organization will undertake a major effort to make this therapy available all over the world through certified homeopathic practitioners. We nevertheless need time to accomplish this enormous project, at least a few years, depending on the enthusiasm of our homeopathic colleagues worldwide. In the Netherlands about 85 homeopaths have been certified as CEASE therapists, and many of them speak English very well. We are already planning how to help children from abroad through Dutch homeopaths who speak English, French and German. Starting in 2010, training programs will be available in English. Homeopaths interested in registering for CEASE training can find the information on our international website www.cease-autism.com. Parents and other interested people can visit the same website to share their experiences, join their national support group and to access information for their homeopath. This website will be constantly updated and give the essential information about this therapy, its availability and about new discoveries. Volunteers in each country will translate this website into their own language and make this information available for everybody.

Can every autistic child be cured with the CEASE therapy? In principle yes, this method works with every child, however there are limitations. I have explained that autism can be reversed because it is a blockage in the brain and not physical damage. But there are cases were autism is combined with diseases involving physical damage to the brain, as in severe epilepsy (e.g. West Syndrome), encephalitis or meningitis. Does it mean that these children will not benefit from the CEASE therapy? Surely they also can benefit from this approach, but complete healing cannot be achieved. Another limitation is that in some cases we cannot determine all the causative factors, which means that we cannot undo all the damage with Isotherapy. Sometimes classical homeopathy or Inspiring Homeopathy can give the helping hand here and finally bring complete healing.

It is my hope that this book will lead to the relief of much emotional pain, both in the autistic children and in their parents, and in all who in any way feel connected to their fate.

Tinus Smits, M.D.

GLOSSARY

ABA: Applied Behavioral Analysis, a mixture of psychological and educational techniques adapted to each individual child, based on the idea that by influencing a response associated with a behavior that behavior will change in the appropriate way.

ASD: Autistic Spectrum Disorder

ascorbate: the salt of ascorbic acid, this makes vitamin C non-acidic and is water-soluble

ascorbyl palmitate: fat-soluble vitamin C

aggravation: a temporary worsening of existing symptoms that can happen as part of the course of homeopathic treatment and healing process, typically followed by improvement.

casein/gluten-free diet: a special diet for autistic children which avoids all casein (milk protein) and gluten (a substance found in grains, especially wheat), which in some cases can improve autistic symptoms.

D6: the homeopathic potency 6x

DAN!: 'Defeat Autism Now', a movement and a protocol attempting to cure autism with nutritional supplements, antifungal (to treat yeast infection in the bowels) and chelation therapy to detoxify heavy metals; must be administered by a physician.

DHA (docosahexanoic acid): one of the omega-3 fatty acids, essential for the membranes of nerve and brain cells; is especially important while the brain is developing during pregnancy and the first 5 years of life.

DMSA: dimercaptosuccinic acid, a substance used to chelate heavy metals (i.e. attach to them in a way that facilitates excretion from the body)

DTaP: vaccination for diphtheria, tetanus, and acellular pertussis (intended to be safer than the whole cell pertussis)

DTP: vaccination for diphtheria, tetanus and pertussis

DTPol: vaccination for diphtheria, tetanus and polio used in the Netherlands

DTPP: Diphtheria, Tetanus, Pertussis and Polio

EPA (eicosapentaenoic acid): one of the omega-3 fatty acids, playing a critical role in immune and inflammatory response; these are anti-inflammatory agents acting in opposition to the omega-6 fatty acids, which are pro-inflammatory agents; EPA is also essential for brain tissues along with DHA.

four-week course: basic treatment of detoxification, repeating a remedy twice a week for four weeks, each week in a different potency, 30C, 200C, 1M, 10M

GMOs (Genetic Modified Organisms): food whose genetic material has been modified

Hep B: vaccination for hepatitis B

Hib: vaccination for haemophilus influenzae type B

HUFA: highly unsaturated fatty acids

intoxication: a state of being ill from toxins, such as from vaccines, medications, environmental chemicals or heavy metals

Isotherapy: a particular form of homeopathy which uses remedies made from the offending substance such as a drug, vaccine or allergen; also known as isopathy.

meconium: the first fecal excretion of a newborn child; if the baby excretes it into the amniotic fluid prior to the delivery, it can cause problems at birth.

metallothionein: one of a family of proteins which protects the body against heavy metals by exchanging zinc for toxic heavy metals (cadmium, mercury, aluminum, etc.). These proteins are synthesized in different crucial parts of the body such as the bowels and brain if sufficient zinc as well as amino acids are present.

MMR: vaccination for measles, mumps and rubella

MSM: methylsulfonylmethane, an organic sulfur compound which is a basic nutrient required for proper functioning of many body functions yet not likely to be adequately supplied in the average diet.

neocortex: the part of the brain responsible for conscious thought, language, spatial reasoning, sensory perception, social-emotional skills and motor commands

Non-Toxic Tumor Therapy: a treatment for cancer developed by the author which combines intensive homeopathic treatment; general detoxification with low potencies to stimulate the liver, digestive system and kidneys; stimulation of the immune system by the administration of vitamins C, E, A, selenium, mushrooms, and other supplements and a healthy diet. This therapy is generally applied together with the regular treatment of surgery, chemotherapy and radiation therapy

orthomolecular medicine: treatment with specific nutritional supplements, often in doses higher than the typical minimum recommended daily doses, the so-called therapeutic dose

otitis media: middle ear infection; **bilateral otitis media:** in both ears at the same time

oxidative stress: caused by free radicals, which are oxygen radicals from the oxygenation process; these free radicals are very reactive and cause damage when not effectively reduced again by anti-oxidants like vitamins and other natural substances.

PDD-NOS: 'pervasive developmental disorder, not otherwise specified.' A catchall diagnosis for children who do not have sufficient symptoms for a diagnosis of autism or of a specific form of pervasive developmental delay or disorder.

Pfeiffer Treatment Center: a facility for nutritional treatment of behavioral disorders and mental illnesses, based on the pioneering work of Carl Pfeiffer of the Princeton Bio Center. *www.hriptc.org*

pharyngitis: sore throat

probiotics: friendly microorganisms that normally live in the intestine and vagina and support healthy function such as digesting food, creating certain vitamins, and resisting the overgrowth of candida; they can be taken in capsule form as supplements, with the best-known form being acidophilus.

PVS, Post-Vaccination Syndrome: chronic ill health resulting from vaccination

Rx: prescription

SonRise therapy: behavioral treatment developed by the Kaufman family for their autistic son. The basic attitude towards the children is love, acceptance, calmness, softness, non-judgment and respectfulness. During the training the child is guiding and by creative and pedagogical interactions new skills are developed.

Specific Carbohydrate Diet: diet which aims to avoid disaccharides and polysaccharides, most sugars, to enter the digestive system; they cause overgrowth of certain bacteria, which leads to a leaky gut syndrome and intoxication of the blood and other systems.

tropical vaccinations: vaccinations for travel to tropical countries; the vaccinations adults are likely to get are typhoid, yellow fever, hepatitis A, sometimes hepatitis B and Rabies, cholera, and a booster of their DTPol.

varicella: chickenpox

vernix caseosa: the protective coating covering a newborn baby's body; this substance has been potentized into a homeopathic remedy for one of the Universal Layers of Inspiring Homeopathy

vital energy: homeopathy's term for the body's healing energy, called *chi* in Traditional Chinese Medicine

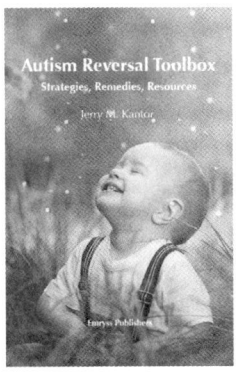

Autism Reversal Toolbox

Strategies, Remedies, Resources

Jerry M. Kantor

In the most comprehensive book to date on the homeopathic treatment of autism, Jerry Kantor introduces a master plan, the Sine Wave Method, offering a diverse range of tools. The toolbox contains (and improves on) the strongest existing approaches plus an expanded arsenal of useful remedies. Clinically successful on a consistent basis, the Sine Wave method also commits to a mission: evolving increasingly potent strategies to understand, eliminate and prevent autism spectrum disorder.

Parents as well as professionals will gain a great deal from this book, as it includes dozens of interventions they can do at home (nutritional supplements, Qi Gong massage, grounding, interactive play) and advice on how to find a homeopath who can treat their autistic child.

DOCUMENTARY ON VACCINATION DAMAGE

AND ITS TREATMENT

'Vaccination Damage Cured!'

In this fascinating and touching documentary Dr. Tinus Smits explains his treatment method, and parents of ill children tell their experience with vaccine damage and the amazing improvements with Dr. Smits' therapy. It includes dramatic before-and-after stories of children cured of vaccination damage, including some of the children whose stories are in this book.

For more information *www.ppdocu.com*

'Freedom of choice in Medicine' The Incurable Cured

(3 cancer patients)

Dr. Tinus Smits has also developed a natural cancer therapy based on homeopathy and supplements. In this documentary, three such patients with "incurable" cancer describe their healing by Dr. Smits' treatment. The documentary further explores the medical establishment's lack of acceptance or even hostility towards such alternative therapies, expressed by the inspector of health. Rogier Hoenders (a psychiatrist) gives his frank opinions about the position of alternative medicines and about why it is so difficult for alternative doctors to do research. The documentary pleads for the patient's freedom to choose therapies that have proven their effectiveness through centuries of use.

For more information *www.ppdocu.com*

FRIENDS OF HOMEOPATHY NEPAL

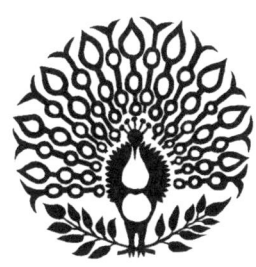 Our philosophy is to share a little bit of our wealth to other people on our earth who don't have the facilities we have in the Western world, not just by giving money, but by helping them to develop themselves. We want to help them to develop cheap and efficient, easily accessible medical care that allows them to stay free and independent. We believe that the best help is to teach them how to practice homeopathy instead of sending homeopathic doctors to treat them. Our philosophy is also to make them responsible for the whole project with a Nepalese staff, medical director, teachers, etc. and not to take over what they can do themselves. We give them the necessary support and provide supervision to make the whole project successful.

Nepal has a harrowing lack of medical doctors and only a small part of the population has access to medical care. We have chosen initially to support the education of Homeopathic Health Assistants (HHA) to make health care available among the poorest, especially in the remote areas of Nepal. This education program of 3 years followed by one year of practical experience in our homeopathic clinic is officially recognized by the Nepalese government. Ten students are educated per year; the poor students get a scholarship (1000€) which is sponsored by gifts from our donors.

Now this school is well underway, our highest goal can be accomplished -- to educate homeopathic doctors at the university level (BHMS). Within one or two years this training can be started.

We only work with volunteers, and the money we collect is used exclusively for scholarships, salaries of teachers and staff, the purchase of materials, construction of a new building for the BHMS faculty and the HHA course.

If you want to support this marvelous project go to: www.homeopathynepal.com and you will be guided to make an easy payment with Paypal or send your money with Paypal directly to: paypal@homeopathynepal.com

The Nepalese people thank you for your generosity.

Stichting Homeopathie Nepal
Vincent van Goghlaan 6
5581 JM Waalre
the Netherlands

For more information see: *www.homeopathynepal.com*